THE RAINBOW DIET

THE RAINBOW DIET AND HOW IT CAN HELP YOU BEAT CANCER

Chris Woollams M.A. (Oxon)

The Rainbow Diet and **Eat a Rainbow**: Copyright © 2008 by Chris Woollams for **icon** magazine, CANCERactive and Health Issues,

The Rainbow Diet – and how it can help you beat cancer:

First Edition published July 2008 by:
Health Issues Ltd
The Elms, Radclive Road, Gawcott, Buckingham, MK18 4JB
Tel: 0203 186 1006
E-mail: enquiries@canceractive.com

Cover design by Jeremy Baker.

ISBN 0-9542968-9-3

Printed in the UK by CPI William Clowes
Beccles NR34 7TL

*'Let your food be your medicine
and let your medicine be your food'*

Hippocrates

Important Notice

This book represents a review and an interpretation of a vast number of varied sources available to anyone on the subject of diet, healthy eating, and cancer, its prevention and possible cure.

Whilst the author has made every effort to ensure that the facts, information and conclusions are accurate and as up-to-date as possible at the time of publication, the author and publisher assume no responsibility.

The author is neither a fully qualified health practitioner nor a doctor of medicine and so is not qualified to give any advice on any medical matters. Cancer (and its related illnesses) is a very serious and very individual disease, and readers must consult with experts and specialists in the appropriate medical field before taking, or refraining from taking, any action.

This book and the advice contained are not intended as an alternative to such specialist advice, which should be sought for accurate diagnosis and before any course of treatment.

The author and the publisher cannot be held responsible for any action, or lack of action, that is taken by any reader as a result of information contained in the text of this book. Such action is taken entirely at the reader's own risk.

This book is dedicated to all the sensible people who know that there is more to life than taking drugs.

PREFACE

Can one book really change your life?

I think The Rainbow Diet can, because I genuinely believe it will give you a much better chance of beating cancer – whether you have it already, or simply want to avoid ever developing it in the first place. Sadly, it is increasingly likely that one in two of us will have to face this hurdle at some point in our lives.

I've written this book because I wanted people to understand how we are ignoring the foods and natural compounds that have protected and corrected us for the last 200,000 years or more. And I wanted to empower people so that they simply understood exactly what a 'Good Diet' entailed, and how it differs from the rag bag of advice you glean from the media, much of which has nothing to do with sensible science but is borne out of politics, ignorance, handed-down mythology or the latest 'fad', whether from the hips of a film star or the lips of a Diet 'expert' who has studied the diet of some distant race living in vastly different circumstances to your own and thinks you should copy it.

In the midst of all this, the real truth is that, all over the world, top scientists have been showing exactly how foods 'work', which ones can help you, and which ones can harm you, often to see their work all but ignored.

Why restrict the message to cancer?

Surely a good diet helps fight heart disease, diabetes and MS and also controls your weight as much as helps fight cancer? This is almost certainly true. And I suppose there is no reason why people cannot use the principles in this book to help them whatever their illness. Certainly a cancer prevention diet would be equally as good as a heart disease or diabetes prevention diet.

But there definitely are some foods that have been shown to have very specific actions in preventing and in restricting cancer and I have focused on those a little more than others. And anyway, the last seven years of my life have been devoted to studying this disease. I don't feel I'm on safe ground commenting on heart disease, but on cancer I genuinely feel I'm an expert.

Back in the spring of 2001 my eldest daughter, Catherine (then 22), developed a malignant brain tumour. Look up glioma on the internet and basically it says, *'You're dead. No hope'.* When we started our research we found that even the mighty UK medical magazine, The Lancet, all but said the drugs were useless.

But, I refused to accept her oncologists offer of, 'Don't worry, we'll give her a good summer'. I read books and covered the internet. I rang experts in orthodox and complementary fields. I talked to people at the boundaries of our cancer knowledge. And I found so much – so very much – information out there, most of which UK oncologists simply do not know exists. For example, there is research on natural compounds that had been shown to have real potential with gliomas: Like echinacea, curcumin, coenzyme Q10, omega-3 and choke berry.

When it came to having **Radiotherapy,** we found that certain natural compounds could improve the success of the treatment, while others could protect the patient from the possible side effects. The MD Anderson Cancer Center in Texas were talking about astragalus, St Thomas' Hospital had conducted limited research on the benefits of isoflavones and selenium; others were using vitamin D.

When it came to having **Chemotherapy** there was suddenly a debate engulfing us about taking antioxidants and whether they would negate the effects of the drugs. Was this really true, or another example of handed-down mythology? I know now that there should be no debate – there is good quality research in the USA – from UCLA, from MD Anderson, from Harvard and others. A number of supplements and the right diet can make your chemotherapy far more effective. (These effects are not confined to chemotherapy for brain tumours. For example with breast cancer patients, clinical trials have shown Tocotrienol vitamin E can reduce the quantity of Tamoxifen you need by 25 per cent, such are its powers to enhance the drug's action.)

The new 'day job'

I'd written a new diet programme for Catherine and she was taking lots of supplements. Importantly everything we did was 'with purpose'. We were not just throwing foods, vitamins and minerals into her with crossed fingers.

After 6 months – the maximum time the doctors had predicted she would live – a scan suggested she was 'All Clear', but with the scarring of the brain tissue no one could be truly certain. Every three months she returned for a further scan, and each was 'clearer'. After two years one of St Thomas' top Doctors suggested I write down what we had found out. And my first book, *"Everything you need to know to help you beat cancer"*, was the result. It sold out after three months!

A Health Company asked me to speak. (Ex-advertising men are always ready to speak on anything!) That led to invitations from the USA, Australia, Japan, Russia, Germany and more.

All the time my knowledge was increasing – I was by now receiving information and newsletters from over 60 cancer centres worldwide. Catherine suggested that we launch a patient-orientated magazine of helpful and highly usable information, and so **icon** (*Integrated Cancer and Oncology News*) was born – at 64 pages in full colour, it is now available free in over 370 UK Cancer Centres, with a conservative estimate of 160,000 readers per quarterly issue. Next it goes into libraries.

We started a cancer charity – CANCERactive – but one with a unique difference: It didn't just tell you about the Orthodox Therapies available, it told you about effective Complementary and Alternative Therapies too; and the latest on possible causes that also might be maintaining the disease. All from the research information I was receiving regularly from top experts.

It's one of the biggest myths of modern medicine: That there's no research evidence for Complementary and Alternative Therapies. There is an enormous amount if you know where to look and have a biochemistry degree to sort the wheat from the chaff. I always knew my Oxford degree wouldn't be wasted – now I have a new, albeit unpaid, job. (All the money from this book, my speeches and everything I do goes to the charity. I don't take a penny.)

Increasing your personal odds of beating diseases

At the speeches, people used always to ask about diet: *'What can I eat to help me beat cancer?'*

I am adamant that the changed diet and selected supplements were a vital factor in helping Catherine survive nearly eight times longer than predicted.

So could we help others? The realisation came at the Cancer Prevention Conference CANCERactive organised. Professor Tony Howell of Christie Hospital, Manchester and one of our patrons, explained that his job was to help women prevent breast cancer returning, in the same or the other breast. But we know that 'good diet' is a significant cancer preventer too – experts will endorse this. So why are people not being told what diet to embrace? I can tell you about natural compounds that reduce inflammation, others that reduce oestrogen levels, others that even kill cancer cells or stop metastasis and others that boost your immune system – and that's for starters. To help people tailor their diet and supplements to their age, situation, type of cancer and individual needs, the charity now offers a programme of Personal Prescriptions available to anyone who fills a form in on our web site.

And increasingly, that is what our charity CANCERactive sets out to do. We aim to provide top-quality research information that empowers you, even inspires you, to build yourself a personal programme, choosing the 'best of the best', and thus increase your odds of beating this disease. Some experts in the USA believe that such an 'integrated' approach can increase your survival odds by over 60 per cent.

For my part, I just try to help people beat cancer.

Eat-to-beat cancer

The first edition of my diet foray was a book called, **The Tree of Life;** it sold out in seven months. We updated it quickly and re-printed. It has now sold over 25,000 copies. I used the symbol of a tree so people could see easily what roots underpinned the 'diet', what supported it and that the volume of the total diet should be in the highly protective branches.

But life moved on rapidly. In speeches I coined the phrase '**The Rainbow Diet**' to show the width of nature's gifts to us including the importance of natural pigments (flavenoids, phenols, antho-cyanins etc) and other food compounds (like vitamin D and fish oils) for your health.

Then came a centerfold in **icon** in the spring of 2006 entitled 'Over *the Rainbow*' – inviting people to take a little daily sunshine, drink clean water and nourish their bodies with a rainbow of foods. We loaded it onto our web site, www.canceractive.com, and it has been one of the five most read pages for two years now.

The Tree of Life was a diet of addition, not deprivation; a book of simple information based on scientific evidence aiming to clear up most of the myths and mumbo-jumbo regularly turned out when the subject of food comes up. It even included a point-scoring system so that you could see how good your diet really was and set yourself some simple, achievable goals.

So we have taken the best of that book, updated it with all the latest scientific research and metamorphosed it into this book: The Rainbow Diet – and how it can help you beat cancer.

Most of all it's an **easy** diet. Easy-to-read, easy-to-understand, easy-to-use. It gives you an understandable plan – including a shopping list.

One final point. I am often asked why I do not include references. The answer is two-fold: I do not write for the scientific or medical worlds but for ordinary folk; people who want to prevent or beat a cancer. And secondly, if you want the references go to our web site, look up Cancer Watch and you will see a synopsis of much of the research produced every month by the world's top cancer centres.

Thank you

So, here we are with **'The Rainbow Diet'**, a book that has evolved from the **'Tree of Life'**. Along the way, many people have helped me. I should like to thank my friend Larry Brooks for kick-starting the project originally, and Lindsey Fealey for all her hard work. Thanks also to Karen Holden and Jane Reynolds, the team at **icon**, including Malcolm, and Ginny Fraser and Madeleine Kingsley, and Phil, the typesetter, for all the proof reading and changes.

Thanks also to Dr Rob Verkerk for helping me with the water chapter, Alan Hopking for his help with herbs, Roger Coghill for his help on melatonin, Gerald Green for his expertise on yeasts and Lawrence Plaskett, Dr Contreras and Charlotte Gerson for spending so much time with me. And thanks to all the research scientists of Cancer Centres from Harvard to Tokyo, and UCLA to Moscow. Your research does matter – it enables people like me to tell the Whole Truth about the benefits of food, and it saves lives.

CONTENTS

SECTION 2 – RE-BUILDING A LIFE

INTRODUCTION
NOURISHMENT AND HEALING

"An apple a day keeps the doctor away.
Especially if well aimed."

(Mark Twain)

Mark obviously had his own theories on diet and doctors. When it comes to nutrition he was probably right on both counts.

The common apple contains, for example, large quantities of potassium but little sodium, good quantities of magnesium, cancer protecting flavenoids, quercitin, polysaccharides and the ability to help promote an alkaline cellular environment. Its pips contain vitamin B-17, whilst the whole apple contains helpful vitamins, enzymes and fibre.

The common doctor, unfortunately, doesn't know too much about any of this. My GP couldn't name a single antioxidant. When I named six for him to write down, he couldn't even spell lycopene.

But I wouldn't wish to criticise doctors for one moment – they are intelligent, caring people who have trained for seven years, and are dedicated to saving our lives. They deserve all the praise we can give them. The people who train them, the ones who set the syllabus and the examinations simply do not ask that they learn much, if anything, about food, diet, nutrition, vitamins, minerals, enzymes and NOURISHMENT.

When talking recently to a newly qualified GP, it transpired that during her seven years training she had spent just one morning on the subject of nutrition – a morning on heart disease.

In the USA, so worried are American Medical Professionals about this very issue that the Physicians Committee for Responsible Medicine (PCRM) is distributing a 900 page guide to medical students in the USA and Canada. This will cover everything from evidence-based information on the role of nutrition in prevention and treatments, to macro- and micro-nutrients for all stages of life. Oh, that we had this initiative in the UK too.

Common contributory factors in heart disease, cancer and

1

diabetes include poor diet, high blood sugar levels, high 'bad' fat consumption, being overweight, smoking, consuming too much salt, lack of exercise, depression and other mental issues like stress and so on. Governments, the press and Health Authorities now harangue us over our modern hedonistic lifestyles: One recent UK report told us that 50 per cent of cancers were our own fault.

Is that really fair? If our Government is quite clear that the roots of the three most common, and increasingly prevalent, diseases lie in poor diet, where are the education programmes on nutrition for school children and for doctors? If our families are not educated in what foods can nourish and protect them, and our doctors are missing an important chunk of the picture when giving us advice on our health, no wonder we are witnessing a crisis in illness levels. The only education we now receive are press and TV advertisements persuading us to eat pizzas and hamburgers!

Constant illness, constant healing

The most curious aspect of modern medicine is that it likes to differentiate between 'prevention' and 'cure'. However, a disease doesn't just happen in one minute; it builds over months or years. And it doesn't stop developing the moment you are officially diagnosed. It is constantly evolving.

The fact is that you are a highly complex 'Chemical Laboratory' with eight trillion chemical reactions happening almost simultaneously. And some inevitably go wrong – throughout the day. So the truth is you actually 'get sick' hundreds of times a day. But the reality is that your body and your immune system constantly correct the problem – they constantly heal you. The likelihood to incur more moments of illness increases the worse your nourishment. The likelihood that your immune system cannot correct and heal you increases the worse your nourishment.

So just as 'illness' moments are constant, so healing is constant and it is aided and abetted by the foods and natural compounds you consume each day.

2

Diets are about addition not deprivation

The truth is that we have evolved to be in harmony with our environments. Go back a thousand years – you ate and drank from your immediate environment. And the foods you ate provided nourishment and also natural compounds, which constantly healed and corrected illnesses. Even though we were surrounded by quite a hostile, microbe-infected environment, we survived and thrived.

Your diet was something that nourished, protected, and corrected. We ate animal fats, became infected with parasites, we ate salt and drank alcohol. But the natural compounds in our vegetables, fruits and herbs boosted, protected, cleansed and killed.

If we eat poor foods – or even no foods – is that likely to nourish, protect and correct?

Using a spectrum of natural compounds to beat cancer

This book is not intended as a detailed scientific tome; it is a normal person's everyday guide to natural compounds and how they can protect and heal you. The intention is that you should be able to put a spectrum of those compounds into your body each week, so that you know that across the average month you have covered all the bases, and done your level best to increase your odds of beating cancer.

In this book I am going to tell you all about the very latest discoveries that will nourish and heal you.

I am going to tell you about beneficial bacteria that will cut up certain high fibre foods in your intestine to produce compounds that will prevent bad cholesterol formation, promote good cholesterol formation and that will actually reduce levels of plaque in the body. If you don't eat high fibre foods you will not get this protection and correction.

I'm going to tell you about mauve pigments that can kill off any pre-cancer cells you make.

I'm going to tell you about an orange spice that helps prevent Alzheimer's and is increasingly studied as a colon-cancer fighter.

And a white bulb that can stop blood supplies forming to tumours.

3

And a natural compound in red grapes that can make you younger and even repair damage to your DNA.

And bright red factors found in raspberries that can stop HPV-infection and heal lesions that can lead to cervical cancer.

And compounds in olive oil and green tea that, according to one American Cancer Center, '*Can stop leukaemia in its tracks*'.

And a common herb that seems to do much the same.

And about certain green foods that contain compounds that can take aggressive oestrogen molecules in your body and down-grade them so that they are less harmful.

And another herb that can make the viruses, bacteria and cancer cells 'light up' on your immune system's radar.

I'll even tell you about half a dozen foods that can reduce inflammation, the precursor to diseases like arthritis and cancer.

And so much more.

Reds and oranges, and yellows and greens, blues, and indigo and violet – all the colours of the rainbow.

And before anyone jumps in to suggest that foods can't 'cure' cancer, I suggest that they consult the Pharmaceutical Companies because right now they are trying to concentrate and patent all manner of natural compounds found in herbs and foods, to make drugs they know have these powers.

You could be eating them right now, with the help of this book. But, make no mistake: By depriving yourself of these natural compounds in your normal diet, you are putting yourself in real danger. By adding them into your normal diet they will protect and correct – nourish and heal.

SECTION 1

KNOWLEDGE IS POWER
BUT, WITH CANCER, IT CAN BE THE DIFFERENCE
BETWEEN LIFE AND DEATH

One day you can read vitamin D is a wonder vitamin, the next there's a problem with it. Then melatonin, the sleep hormone, helps defeat breast cancer – but it is illegal to sell it in the UK. The Government wants you to avoid fats, salt and sugar – yet hospitals produce booklets for patients having chemotherapy telling them to eat cheeseburgers, sugared buns and milkshakes! Dairy may be harmful if it is a Tuesday, vitamin E if it's a Friday. My doctor says *'You don't need supplements if you eat a balanced diet'* but then he tells me he's never studied nutrition. The Government and Cancer experts tell me to *"Eat five portions of fruit and vegetables a day, don't smoke and stay out of the sun. And remember 50 per cent of cancers are your own fault because of your lifestyle'*. I wonder what the other 50 per cent is and who is in charge of that! And anyway, isn't sunshine good for me?

No wonder we're all confused.

CHAPTER 1

WHAT IS CANCER – AND HOW COULD DIET POSSIBLY HELP?

My cousin Lindsey Fealey, who was CEO of our charity at the time, was 'manning a stand' for CANCERactive at the nurses conference in York a few years ago. Two rather plump nurses wandered over. One picked up a copy of the first edition of the *Tree of Life*, opened it, then a few seconds later tossed it back on the table hitting Lindsey in the face with the words, *'How could anyone be stupid enough to think diet could beat cancer?'*

Cancer is primarily a modern disease. An American research study of 7,000 years of skeletons in Croatia showed the first signs in bones dating from less than 100 years ago. We do know that there were illnesses called cancers as long ago as Ancient Egypt, Greece and Rome – Aloe Vera was used to treat skin cancers; Hippocrates actually treated patients with a special soup and enemas. But cancer in any volume was almost unheard of before the Industrial Revolution.

The World Health Organisation denotes poor diet, toxins (including smoking) and infection/disease as the prime causes.

Why are we so concerned about cancer?

Because you are very likely to develop it.

UK cancer levels have doubled over the last 30 years to a current annual figure of 320,000 (including skin cancer, which is usually omitted from the total figure). They are forecast to double again in the next 20 years. At the moment about 1.5 million people are living with cancer in the UK and, whatever you may read or hear from the media, it is a clear fact that more people die every year from cancer now than ten, fifteen or twenty years ago. We are not 'beating cancer'. To claim otherwise ignores the hard facts.

One in two men living today will develop cancer, one in three women. And estimates, (for example from leading Canadian scientists in 2006), suggest we are heading to one in two people overall.

Now let's get back to the main question!

Textbook theories

Your body is in a state of constant change. Old cells die, new cells replace them. Every moment of your day, your cells are copied at different rates depending upon the tissue, but always in an orderly, 'disciplined' manner. There can be millions of cell divisions every day.

Sometimes something goes wrong. For example:

- You may lack something important to that copying process, for example folic acid.
- Or something 'nasty' (the technical term is a 'carcinogen') like a chemical toxin may interfere with this copying process.
- Or something may block the genetic code's ability to send out the correct message.

Damaging your genetic blueprint is called a mutation; text books might point to **Direct** exposure to X-Rays, or radiation, even drugs as examples of causes. But it doesn't have to be an external factor. You may have heard of the term 'free radicals'. These are 'toxic' molecules with imperfect, 'sticky' ends and they will happily rip bits off any nearby molecule starting a chain reaction inside a cell.

For thousands of years our wonderful immune systems have protected us from all this, identifying, neutralising and taking away rogue cells.

But what if certain factors have weakened your immune system? These could be **Indirect** factors that do not actually cause a rogue cell, but nonetheless do allow one to beat the defences and start its progress towards become a fully fledged cancer. For example the immune system might be weakened in such a way that it cannot 'see' the rogue cell.

And so the text book theory of cancer developed.

Other issues were identified – antioxidants could neutralise the free-radicals; the immune system worked best when it was in a slightly alkaline environment. But the principle was simple: A rogue cell developed and beat the system.

Breakthrough thinking – stem cells

In November 2004 Professor Wang and his team from British Columbia presented a new theory based on their research. They claimed the text books 'would need to be re-written'.

When conducting research on stomach cancer, Wang observed that after localised inflammation had occurred, stem cells rushed from the bone marrow to the area of the stomach wall in trouble. But instead of converting into new stomach lining cells, they stayed as stem cells growing uncontrollably. Wang observed that this was due to the effects of localised oestrogen, the female sex hormone.

What are stem cells? They are the cells of the foetus – elementary basic cells that can be converted by the body (the technical term is differentiated) into any cell required. In fact, you have stem cells throughout your life; you need new basic cells at all times – or how would you make new eye cells, or kidney cells or liver cells?

In fact Wang's 'breakthrough' was 98 years out of date – the theory had already been put forward by John Beard, a Scottish Embryologist.

Some breast cancers and brain tumours are known to arise from stem cells in this way.

The implications of this theory are enormous: For example, an important one would be that your immune system wouldn't recognise these as rogue cells – after all, they contain your normal DNA. And it is certainly the case that in some cancers your immune system seems almost powerless.

Oestradiol

Every cell has receptor sites on its surface. Chemical messages arrive at these sites and activate events inside the cell. Certain receptor sites receive messages from the oestrogen family of hormones. One family member, called oestradiol, is very dangerous when it alights on the receptor sites and can cause havoc inside the cell. Fortunately, there is a 'sister hormone', oestrone, that is about forty times less powerful.

Plants have similar hormones, called phytoestrogens, which are thankfully far less aggressive still and are actually known to be able to bind to these receptor sites and therefore block oestradiol from taking up these dangerous positions. If only diet could convert dangerous oestradiol into its weaker sister, or perhaps find a way of blocking the receptor sites.

When oestradiol does alight on a normal cell, various biochemical changes are noted inside the cell. Levels of sodium increase, levels of potassium fall. The cell becomes more acidic, it uses less oxygen and it produces less energy.

Several cancers have been observed to be 'oestrogen' driven. It fuels the fire in most breast cancers, most stomach and bowel cancers, some lung cancers, most prostate cancers and many womb cancers

Low magnesium/high sodium

But you don't need oestradiol to produce these effects.

Recent US research showed that 40 per cent of Americans are deficient in magnesium. This is very worrying. Magnesium is essential as it is involved in operating a pump on the cell wall. This pump keeps high levels of potassium inside the cell, and keeps sodium levels low. If the pump doesn't work well and/or if you flood your body with salt (sodium), then the cells and their power stations (called mitochondria) become poisoned. Yes, they can run on sodium, but 200,000 years of evolution has simply meant that they run much better on potassium.

In fact, we are Potassium People. It's what makes us work properly. Our cells and our immune systems.

If too much sodium is present, the normal twenty-plus step energy production system (the Krebs cycle) becomes less efficient and starts to slow down, drawing less oxygen in and producing less energy. It also produces waste sodium salts, which are much more acid than potassium ones. So the cell starts to become more acidic, and that further impairs the chemical reactions and the inflow of oxygen. Even less energy is produced and yet more sodium salts. You are on a downward spiral.

10

When the level of energy production falls below a certain figure (think of the power station as a battery) the p53 repair gene switches off, but the genes that make the cell divide *(ras* genes) need far less power and still operate. Cells with no repair system but dividing uncontrollably in the absence of oxygen? A cancer in the making.

Clearly there are diet factors behind this route.

Infection

The World Health Organisation believes about 15 per cent of cancers are 'caused' by infection – viruses, bacteria, microbes, yeasts, and parasites. Each is really a parasite under a different name. They can rob you of nourishment, cause inflammation (many cancers have a prior step of inflammation), produce toxins and even carcinogens. And several experts think the estimate of 15 per cent is way too low. Could you have a parasite?

Your diet can actually give you one – sushi and improperly washed exotic fruits would be two examples. But your diet can also take one away – there are natural compounds like garlic, chilli and cinnamon that feature in the diets of certain populations and these can help·kill off a yeast or microbe; and the development of a thriving immune system anyway will give you a much greater protection and resistance.

Many ways to develop cancer

Would you like a few more options? A biological clock protein can repair DNA damage, as can the proteins from several genes. Reduce their presence and you're in trouble. Other genes help the immune system recognise a 'rogue' cell, but sometimes they get turned off. A protein uPA, found by Copenhagen University, is required to spread cancer and cancer cannot spread without its presence. Under certain conditions you may start to make this protein.

I will stop here. I could give you several other possible ways a cancer cell might come about. The main point is that there may be many, many ways a cancer 'rogue' cell can develop and get through your defences. Why should there be just one? And the truth is that the scientists know this too. <u>There is no single textbook programme for the development of every cancer.</u>

Your cancer is as individual as you are

I'm not just saying that all 'types' of cancer (breast, colon, prostate etc) are different – there are over 200 types of cancer, anyway. I am saying that beyond this, there may be many ways you can develop a breast cancer or a brain tumour. The fact that orthodox medicine has now acknowledged that there are oestrogen positive, or progesterone positive, or HER-2 positive, or now stem cell breast cancers indicate this as well. And scientists are already developing a range of drugs for breast cancer to deal with these different sub-groups. Sadly, they are a long way away from doing so with other cancers.

I'd go a step further – I believe your cancer is as individual as you are. Of course, there are 'more common' formations, but I really can't agree to 'one size fits all', and this is one of the reasons, I don't think that there will even be a single wonder drug. And oncologists already know this too.

Cancer is a whole body disease

But there are some common factors: For example, if you take the blood of someone with cancer and put it under a microscope you will usually observe two things.

- The red cells are clumped together – meaning there are lowered levels of blood oxygen.
- The white cells are static – meaning the immune system is weak.

Also, the liver of cancer patients is almost always toxic, not damaged but debilitated, poisoned by the effects of the cancer and its causes. And your liver controls your whole body – from its ability to be detoxified, to the strength of the immune system to the energy production systems.

This is important because it suggests that whilst a cancer tumour may well be localised, the conditions that caused it and its effects are present throughout the body. Cancer is a disease of the whole body – and you have to treat it as such.

12

Cancer cells are different

All cancer cells do, in fact, resemble stem cells in their behaviour. Stem cells are often termed 'very primitive' in that, as I said before, they are basic cells not yet differentiated into anything specific. Because you need lots of them as a 'store of replacement parts' for your body, they divide rapidly. Cancer is defined in the dictionary as 'An uncontrolled growth of cells derived from normal tissues'

Stem cells do not die, they merely move on to other cell forms. Cancer cells do not die, they just multiply.

Cancer cells, however, do not use the lengthy Krebs cycle for energy production – instead they use a short fermentation process that does not require oxygen and generates their energy by burning glucose. Otto Warburg won a Nobel Prize in 1931 for telling the world this, and that getting oxygen to a cancer cell could bring about its downfall.

Cancer cells need higher levels of glucose to produce the same amount of energy as a normal cell, because fermentation is a less efficient process than the Krebs cycle. And they need even more glucose still because they are dividing much more rapidly than normal cells.

One result of this frenetic activity is that cancer cells need iron, and often the cancer patient is anaemic.

The waste product they produce is a form of lactic acid – the cousin of the acid that gives sportsmen cramp. This can only be detoxified in the liver, where it is converted back into glucose, which passes back round the body to feed the tumour – Alien has taken over the mother ship.

This shorter energy-producing cycle of the cancer cell is quite different from that in a normal cell in other ways too: For example it even has its own unique set of enzymes not found in normal healthy cells. Scientists are actually working on drugs that can target these unique enzymes – but as we shall see, some foods are already known to uniquely target these enzymes and destroy them.

Cancer cells do not normally die. One exception is when they are exposed to heat (hyperthermia). This may be caused by external treatment – but, again, some natural compounds found in foods can promote the condition in cells.

So – how can anyone think diet could help beat cancer?

I hope this brief foray into the world of biochemistry has not bored you. I did it for a reason:

I hope you can now see that any cancer – your cancer – might have come about in any number of ways. It is as individual as you are. And it is also a systemic, all-over-body disease.

And as I went through the options could you see how diet might play a role?

As I go through this book I will show you how a good diet and natural compounds can help by:

- **Providing important factors to perfect DNA copying**
- **Providing important factors to correct DNA mis-copying**
- **Avoiding excesses of factors that increase free radicals**
- **Providing more antioxidants to neutralise free radicals**
- **Removing the toxic chemicals and heavy metals from your body and cells**
- **Boosting your immune system and helping it 'see' rogue cells**
- **Keeping your cells and immune system alkaline**
- **Avoiding parasite and microbial infection**
- **Minimising pathogens in the blood stream**
- **Reducing inflammation – a precursor of many cancers**
- **Preventing a blood supply to the developing tumour**
- **Lowering aggressive oestradiol levels**
- **Keeping blood and cellular oxygen levels up**
- **Strengthening your liver, and therefore your immune system**
- **Increasing your pancreatic enzyme production**
- **Killing cancer cells**
- **Increasing survival rates**

These are just 17 examples – it could have been more! The fact is that science has shown, rather unsurprisingly I suppose, **there are natural compounds that can have a significant effect in each of the many cancer stages.**

Please be clear – this statement is very different to claiming a food or a natural compound is a 'cure' for cancer. No natural compound, to my knowledge, can be honestly said to work on **all of the development stages** of cancer. But then certainly no drug should claim this either.

- For example, there is good research that isoflavones and garlic can stop the blood supply forming for tumours. But there is little evidence they can attack and kill a cancer cell or stop it firing off secondaries.
- For example, there are a number of compounds – from salicylin to omega 3 – which can reduce inflammation, but there is little evidence they can help the immune system recognise a rogue cell and kick it out.

Cancer isn't an item – it's a process

And that leads me to another important conclusion that can be drawn from this little look at the life and times of a cancer. I have shown how there can be many 'types' of cancer which have developed in different ways. But more than that, a cancer can be present in any number of stages – rogue cell, tumour formation and metastasis being just three.

So you should not think of cancer as a 'single item' – it is a complex, multi-step, multi-stage process. It's not an ant you can tread on. It's a complex chain of events and you need a width – a package – of activities that can tackle it.

I only gave you a taster above. John Boik of The MD Anderson Cancer Center in Texas estimates that there are 20 stages of cancer – and you may have any number of them in your body at any one time.

Just as I don't think that there will ever be a 'magic bullet' to kill all the different 'types' of cancer, I also don't think there will be one to kill the cancer in all the many stages it might be in within your body. It is simply too much to ask of one drug, one natural compound or one herb. But I do genuinely believe you could have a number of selected natural compounds and herbs each of which tackled different stages of the cancer formation and existence and so worked synergistically to tackle the whole job. And by the end of this book I sincerely hope you will agree.

Boik's theory is contained in his book called 'Natural Compounds in Cancer Therapy'. There he looked at over 4,000 major research studies on natural compounds – and that was in 2001. There would be triple that number nowadays!!

And from this he assigned various natural compounds (including foods, herbs and supplements) against the twenty stages, in terms of their proven scientific abilities.

Now, I'm not going to frighten you in this book with the biochemistry of how each foodstuff fights each step. I'm not a professor talking to scientists at a symposium. I'm a knowledge-able layman trying to help people who want to beat cancer, build a picture of what foods should be in their diet. And that's what I will do.

But I think that the crux of this whole chapter is an understanding that cancer is:

- A disease that can have many drivers – it's as individual as you are.
- A disease that can have many stages – it's a process not an item.

And natural compounds have been proven in history and increasingly in the latest research to be able can tackle each and every facet of both of these.

Yes, I'm stupid enough to think that diet could help beat cancer.

CHAPTER 2
TOXIC BODIES

We receive a vast number of telephone calls, emails and enquiries into the CANCERactive offices from people newly diagnosed with cancer. In 95 per cent of cases, it takes about two minutes, often less, to see what is wrong – what caused the cancer: Most people are both **Toxic,** and **Nutritionally Deficient**.

Some aspects of 'Toxicity' may be caused by poor diet. Obviously, addressing the issue of poor diet is the prime purpose of this book and we will cover it in due course. But there are other causes of toxicity which I need to cover here, especially as I'm sure most people would assume diet had no role to play in helping overcome these 'non-diet induced problems' – and they'd be wrong!

Much of this toxicity is down to this modern world of ours – and it's getting worse.

Drugs

Some people in the medical profession like to tell you that modern drugs have all been through extensive clinical trials to prove their efficacy and safety. Sadly, they are deluded. Only about 15 per cent of the drugs available in the UK today have been through a clinical trial. Even then, the latest clinical trials quantify the benefits but rarely quantify the side effects. The great white hope of more tightly targeted drugs with less side effects also seems an illusion. The Lancet Oncology magazine reported on the problems of high levels of side effects when testing new monoclonal antibodies in 2007. We've all read of 'Elephant man' drug tests and deaths caused by Vioxx, with associated scandals. We are not deluded.

More worrying is the increasing volume of drugs consumed. While one drug may have been through a clinical trial, rarely – if ever – have combinations. Someone on heart medication may be taking others to prevent nausea and side effects. They then get a cold and cough and take paracetamol, antibiotics and cough mixture. According to Dr Stern at the New York Presbyterian

Hospital, it is not uncommon for people over 65 years of age to take more than 6 or even 10 drugs at one time. He should know. So alarmed was he at the increasing level of hospital admissions he joined other doctors in coining a new disease, 'Polypharmacy' – illness due to a cocktail of drugs.

Polypharmacy now accounts for 28 per cent of all hospital admissions in the US. These have more than tripled in the last seven years – as has the death rate from the disease. It now lies behind heart disease, but ahead of cancer in the mortality charts.

Drugs are tested on fit, healthy young to middle aged people. Two thirds of them are used by the over 65 age group whose biological systems are weaker and less able to deal with the toxins.

But don't think this is something beyond your own personal world. US Medical web sites claim cancers like kidney cancer can be caused by painkillers. In **icon** we covered research that showed taking paracetamol with coffee can cause liver damage! How many times have you seen someone do that?

The truth is that all drugs are toxic; all drugs have (even minor) side effects. And this includes the contraceptive pill, HRT (the alarming figures are on our web site) and synthetic vitamin pills too.

Worryingly, three quarters of the Personal Prescriptions I receive come from people who have had an illness for six or more years and have been taking a cocktail of drugs – for diabetes, thyroid, intestinal problems etc. Did they ever think to go to a naturopath or nutritionist? Do they and their doctor understand that taking drugs for six years may merely be covering up an underlying problem which could have/should have been addressed? Leaving it, and adding immune weakening drugs just makes matters worse.

We had one lady develop oesophagael cancer – she'd been on a stomach drug for 10 years. On the web it said quite clearly that the drug 'should not be prescribed for more than six months'. We asked her doctor what he thought might have caused her cancer. His reply? *'Just bad luck'*.

Finally, a recent study showed that 524 drugs available in the USA had actually been manufactured in China – a country that has had more than its fair share of criticism over poor quality controls. Many more are made in other 'cheaper' production countries. Questions asked of the American drug approval organisation, the FDA, produced a response that less than three per cent of overseas drug production was ever monitored or safety checked. One wonders what percentage of UK administered drugs are safety checked, or have their production monitored, their factories visited.

Chemicals

One million tonnes of chemicals were made in the world in 1946. Now the figure is 500 million tonnes. Apart from drugs and pesticides, where does it all go?

In *'Everything you need to know to help you beat cancer'* I go into more detail. But the answer starts with your home. The atmosphere in an American home has been shown to be more toxic than standing in Times Square, New York.

Household cleaners, bleaches, bathroom toiletries, shampoos, hair dyes, perfumes and so on contain chemicals that can disrupt your hormones, or chemicals that can poison you and are actually banned in other countries of the world. A number of these chemicals are proven carcinogens – even Teflon is not beyond criticism. Nor are glues for carpet, ceiling tiles and chipboard nor lead in old paint. According to the US Environmental Protection Agency 1,500 hazardous substances are found in the average American home.

In 2007, Euro MP's voted in favour of banning certain everyday chemicals like formaldehyde – it is already banned in Sweden and Japan. The Commissioners were lobbied by vested interests and did not ratify the bill, instead proposing a re-think and it has gone back to the drawing board.

Europe is not alone in this stalled legislation. There are 80,000 chemical registered in the USA, 15,000 in daily use and Federal Law does not require chemical companies to even review potential hazards! In 2005 there were 35 bills against hazardous chemical in the US legislature – all failed. California has announced it is going to 'go it alone' in terms of regulating chemicals in the state. The latest news involved finding hermaphrodite fish (fish with both sexual organs) off the coast, thought to be the result of chemical waste passing down the rivers. Enough is enough, says California. We'll see.

There are several studies from Friends of the Earth showing that of 78 harmful chemicals, most of us now have between 25 and 49 in our bodies. And it is getting worse. Another of their studies reviewed levels in grandparents and grandchildren, finding find twice as many in the youngsters.

Pesticides, fertilisers and herbicides

To complete the chemical trilogy, there are pesticides, fertilisers and herbicides. We know that farmers have higher rates of certain leukaemias and myeloma; and incidence of leukaemia is increasing in homes next to golf courses in Australia. Children in households using garden and household pesticides have higher rates of certain cancers and there's even a link to flea collars! IARC have pointed a finger at nitrates and nitrites in fertilisers – with links to stomach, oesophagael and brain cancers.

In the UK Government Ministers responsible for pesticides and safety (DEFRA) requested a Royal Commission on Environmental Pollution. Despite conclusions that criticised existing policies, the Government has refused to recognise health risks as a result of spraying agricultural crops. Pesticides were not even mentioned in the 2004/5 White Paper on cancer.

Campaigners are now actually taking the UK Government to the High Court. However, the UK Government view is in direct contrast to that of the EU, who on 12th July 2006 stated that *'Long term exposure to pesticides can lead to serious disturbances to the immune system, sexual disorders, cancers, sterility, birth defects, damage to the nervous system and genetic damage'*. If that's not cause for concern, then I'm not sure what is!

EMF's

The mobile phone and brain tumour controversy may well be reaching its end game as the WHO/Interphone worldwide study already has some researchers in some countries jumping the gun, and publishing their research in advance of the total results. All researchers to date are saying there could well be problems with long term (over 10 years) usage. Australian experts are the latest to agree with experts in Sweden and Norway on this matter.

But more worrying is the bigger picture – the toxicity in our bodies caused by 'electrosmog'. 1,500 phone masts have actually been pulled down in Taiwan, such were the health concerns. They are not the only country waking up to the threat. Worse, WiFi has absolutely no proper research on its safety, and small scale studies have even indicated that it might be more dangerous than direct beams from phone masts. Yet hotels, airports, apartment blocks, offices, the London Underground and even schools and hospitals rush to install it.

Computer screens, TV's in your bedroom and natural fault lines give off these EMF's and there are now clear research links (for example, between power cables and child leukaemia) with cancer.

As we will see later, these effects may not be direct genetic changing effects, but more likely effects causing a weakening of the immune system. One way this can happen is through melatonin depletion. Melatonin is a hormone most normally produced about 90 minutes after you fall asleep. It puts you into a deeper sleep. Its levels affect various other hormones, regulating oestrogen levels and the level of IGF-1, a hormone that increases cell division. And it is a powerful antioxidant. Now IARC have endorsed US research that shows melatonin depletion is carcinogenic.

EMF's are known to cause melatonin depletion.

Negating the damage - the amazing role diet can play

The question you must be asking yourself is, 'With all this going on around me what chance have I got?'

The answer is, 'A really good one'.

It is true SOME toxins cause genetic damage, but only a very few cancers come about in this way. This **Direct** attack produces rogue DNA, but, as a cause of cancer, this is not as great as people might suggest, largely because most such changes usually result in gobble-de-gook being produced, which will be mopped up by your immune system.

In more cases the toxins don't change the actual DNA structure but disrupt the chemical messages that it directs – for example, certain proteins or hormones. This may result in certain essential chemicals being over- or under-produced. And these can have a huge and damaging effect on the body.

Where meaningful genetic changes do occur, it is hard to imagine how diet could possibly reverse (i.e. re-alter) those genetic changes. However you could imagine that some of these genetic mutation cancers or damaged message delivery systems might have their progress halted, or their effects minimised by diets which, for example, compensated for excesses or deficiencies caused by the genetic changes.

Pie in the sky? I can tell you that there are a number of natural compounds that can make a difference and can compensate for these imbalances – the research is very new.

Don't just believe me – the Dana-Faber Cancer Institute have stated that there is no reason why the effects of cancer cannot be reversed. In cloning experiments with mice and melanoma, they concluded that, **whilst the body could not re-alter rogue DNA to make it normal again, the effects could be turned off and neutralised**. Thus, they concluded, **malignancy was not the inevitable effect of a cancer cell**.

Some people may feel cancer runs in their family and they have little chance of beating it. Firstly it is true that you may have an hereditary genetic issue, but again this is not as widespread as some people suggest. It occurs in less than seven per cent of the population, although it is true that people with these problems seem to be particularly affected by toxins and chemicals. However, a Swedish Epidemology study showed that identical twins who lead different lifestyles can have very different risk levels – so there is much you can do with your diet to minimise the risks.

By far largest group of people have not been 'Directly' genetically poisoned anyway – with them, toxins have an **Indirect** effect in the cancer process – for example, by weakening the immune system, by poisoning the cells, or by feeding dangerous hormones which may stimulate and maintain it. And all of these really can be addressed and corrected by a good diet.

Where the changes are not structural, few of the toxins cannot be eliminated from your body, and diet can have a significant effect. For example:

- Pesticide research with children shows that switching to an organic diet 'washed' out key pesticides within 5 days.
- Heavy metals that are cumulative can be tackled by changes to the diet. Selenium is known to replace certain heavy metals from tissues; chlorella and spirulina can displace others.
- Beneficial bacteria have been shown in clinical trials to break down toxic oestrogenic and nitrosamine compounds, and bind to heavy metals to aid their excretion.
- Dangerous oestrogenic products – both human and chemical – have been shown in research to be broken down and neutralised by certain natural compounds like indoles
- Where toxins have caused mineral imbalances in the cells leading to acid cells, high potassium, high magnesium and low sodium diets have been shown to return cells to their healthy normal alkaline states.
- Even dangerous chemicals like dioxins have been shown to have their effects neutralised by certain foods and natural compounds, as we shall see.

So already we are building a picture that even where external factors like chemicals or EMF's may have significantly contributed to your cancer, research shows there are many things you can do in your diet to increase your personal odds of survival.

This is nothing new. Your body, its immune system and its little helpers – the beneficial bacteria in your intestine – have spent 200,000 years helping you kick out unwanted toxins using certain everyday foods as catalysts or carriers. For example, when beneficial bacteria break down oestrogenic chemicals they use plant indoles to help them cause destructuring, and plant lignans to carry the by-products out of the body. The question you need to ask yourself is, *'Do I eat enough of the everyday foods that contain indoles and lignans, and do I have enough beneficial bacteria to complete the job?'*

CHAPTER 3
ATOMIC MAN

Can you really change your cells?

The fully healthy body works in a state of balance and harmony. The unhealthy body is in a state of imbalance and disharmony.

This balance and harmony is both internal – through all your hormone, nervous and enzyme systems, from your brain right to the power stations in your breast or prostate cells – and external – in your inter-relationship with you localised, immediate environment, like the air you breathe, the water you drink, the flowers and the foods growing in your back garden.

Some civilisations believed that an illness in one person was a reflection of the strength of the whole tribe. Modern Governments would do well to study this.

At least 99 per cent of you and me is air, although, to look at each of us, I admit it is hard to imagine. Every molecule in your body is made of atoms and these are simply electrons spinning around a nucleus of neutrons and protons. Both electrons and neutrons are infinitesimally small particles, and between them, relatively speaking, are huge spaces or air masses. Think in terms of the earth, the sun and the moon, and you will understand the massive air gaps relative to the small 'solid' masses in an atom.

Atoms attract and repel other atoms. They are little electronic forces each with their own magnetic field. Too many of one atom might completely overwhelm the presence of another and prevent it from doing its job. It might simply displace it from its position in a molecule, and thus might stop the molecule working properly and helping other molecules work properly.

Building the correct molecules with the correct atoms makes for a body in harmony and balance with all its systems working perfectly. Obtaining the right numbers of atoms for your body is very important. Insufficient of the right ones, or too many of the wrong atoms will lead to illnesses.

This is not just a mathematical and practical issue. It is an energetic issue. If you have the wrong atoms and molecules in your breast cells you will also experience the wrong electronic and magnetic forces in those tissues. Since the Russian scientist Kirlian, we have been able to see the damage caused to our electronic fields around our body by excesses or deficiencies of minerals, and by illnesses. Interestingly, US scientists showed that our electronic fields (or auras) around our body 'become sick first'. And this is already being used in a variety of new diagnostic tools.

These electronic forces are very powerful. They affect and are affected by all manner of external atoms and their electronic fields. Recent research showed that little lizards climb up walls because each of their toes has a thousand minute hairs under them. The molecular fields of these hairs actually inter-react with the molecular fields of the atoms in the wall and 'hold', being released by a nervous impulse sent from the brain when the animal wants to move. Such electronic interactions can make and break hundreds of times per second.

So where are the limits of your body? Certainly the electronic forces do not stop at your skin. The influence on your body of radiation from a mobile phone, power cables, WiFi, microwaves and X-rays is easy to understand.

Everyone has the power to change

It is easy to see how you might poison your metabolism quite quickly. But it is also easy to see how your recovery is equally possible. Clearly:

- **You have the power to change your own internal atoms.**
- **And you have the power to control how many 'good' atoms you have.**
- **And you have the power to stop negative external influences, and to build positive ones.**

Every day you exchange millions of atoms with your environment. Every time you breathe or eat or drink, and even through your skin. So much so that **every 90 days the great majority of the body's tissues have atoms that are completely new to the body.**

You are 'Atomic Man' – a truly bionic being.

26

Four atoms in the health of your cells and immune system

The sodium-potassium balance

Strictly speaking, salt is sodium chloride. It doesn't matter whether it comes from the sea or from mountains – it is sodium chloride.

You may hear the word 'salts'. This is something completely different. All manner of compounds are salts, like carbonates, nitrates, bicarbonates, sulphates of many atoms like sodium, magnesium, aluminium etc.

Moreover, while salt contains sodium, not all sodium is consumed in salt. We ingest sodium as table salt (sodium chloride), preservative salt in meats and other foods (sodium nitrate, sodium nitrite); or taste enhancing salt (like monosodium glutamate).

Whichever way we take our sodium, the average individual in the West consumes much, much more than they need. So much more that it is making them ill. As animals in the wild, hundreds of thousands of years ago we ate virtually no salt. Indeed, we had to go to a salt 'lick' just to get some. By the Middles Ages salt was still a rarity and had become a currency to barter with. Hence the origins of the word salary from the Latin word *'salarium'; 'sal'* being the word for salt. Salt had its place, but largely as a preservative for food stored for the winter months. From all this I could easily construct an argument that the maximum sodium intake should be around one gram per day in the cold climate of the UK. Yet the Food Standards Agency (FSA) still says six grams for adults and three for children, with no detailed rationale given. Worryingly, eight grams is a more usual Western consumption, whilst the average New Yorker consumes about eight kilogrammes per year or over twenty grams per day! And that is an average figure!

In February 2004 the US Institute of Medicine published a report stating that healthy 19–50-year-olds should consume 1.25 grams of sodium per day, much nearer to the figure I have suggested. Even allowing for the weight of the chloride or nitrite, this would yield an upper 'salt' limit of around 5 grams maximum. They note that 95 per cent of American males and 75 per cent of American females exceed this figure.

icon reported on new Japanese research that showed people who ate 12–15 grams of 'salt' per day on average doubled their risk of stomach cancer (*British Journal of Cancer*, February 2004).

Excess sodium has a devastating effect on all cellular membranes and inhibits the correct flow of essential elements into the cell. To that end it affects everything from your brain cells, to your immune cells, and virtually all the normal and healthy metabolic processes in every cell of your body.

It is impossible to talk about sodium without talking about potassium – they are opposing forces. Potassium is essential to the healthy workings inside your cells. Without it the cell becomes imbalanced and unhealthy. The easiest way to think of this is that sodium should largely work outside the cell, while potassium works inside the cell. Too much sodium stops potassium getting into a cell and, worse, actually causes the kidneys to expel it from the body as a whole.

If excess sodium gets inside the cell, it will prevent the proper action of potassium and will result in serious harm. Excess sodium poisons cells and, as we mentioned earlier, their power stations. Over thousands of years, our power stations, or mitochondria, have evolved to use potassium. It could have been anything – that's evolution for you – but it has turned out to be potassium. This is what makes them run smoothly, and potassium hydroxide, one of the main waste products produced, is alkaline.

If sodium displaces the potassium in the power stations, they will still work, but just not as well. The chemical reactions falter, the cell works inefficiently. Sodium waste products are produced and these are more acid than the potassium ones so the system becomes more acidic and yet more poisoned, drawing in less oxygen and producing less power, and the next cycle produces even more sodium salts and makes the cell even more acid, drawing in even less oxygen and producing even less energy. It's a vicious downward spiral and the cell is on its way to being a typical oxygen-free, restricted reaction, low powered cancer cell.

If you want healthy cells your dietary intake of these two atoms should significantly favour potassium, about five to one over sodium. If you consume a gram of sodium today, can you really consume five of potassium? I doubt it. Just look at these figures for guidance.

Prime sources of **stressful sodium** are (approximately in milligrams):

Salt (1 teaspoon)	2000
Cheese, processed (100 gms)	1200
Cheese spread (100 gms)	1100
Oxo cube (1)	1030
Bacon (1 rasher)	1000
Chicken nuggets (6)	1000
Corned beef (100 gms)	1000
Soy sauce (1 tablespoon)	1000
Gravy and sauces (100 gms)	1000
Cornflakes (100 gms)	1000
White bread (4 slices)	900
Baking soda (1 teaspoon)	820
French fries, salted (1 portion)	750
Cheddar cheese (100 gms)	600
Sausage (1 medium)	500
MSG (1 teaspoon)	500
Baked beans, canned (100 gms)	500
Pie casing (1)	500
Cottage cheese (100 gms)	450
Soup, canned	450
Fish, canned	450
Peanuts (100 gms)	420
Fish fingers (100 gms)	400
Spaghetti hoops, canned (100 gms)	400
Biscuits (100 gms)	375
Baking powder (1 teaspoon)	350
Crisps (2 packets)	350
Butter or margarine, salted (2 tablespoons)	250

So you can see stressful sodium is found in certain categories of foods: preserved meats and sausages, condiments (from tomato ketchup to soy sauce), canned foods, breakfast cereals, bread (white or wholemeal), biscuits and cakes, all baked flour products, fast food, crisps and peanuts. Worst are preserved foods and processed foods, while a Chinese meal can give you a whopping 14 gms of the stuff.

Obviously fish, particularly shellfish, contain sodium (but nowhere near the levels of bread or fast foods) and even beer and fizzy soft drinks contain quite high levels of sodium to enhance the taste!

An excess of sodium is debilitating. Apart from its potential disruptive and even cancer-inducing effects inside the cell, it affects the water balance of the body and causes stress, fatigue and even depression.

Perky potassium is highly corrective of this. Apart from its control of the energy production in our cellular power stations, it affects crucially our protein and DNA synthesis. It helps in brain function, nerve transmission and muscle tone and is anti-ageing, whilst excess sodium ages tissues.

So it's not just about cutting sodium consumption. It is about consuming the right quantities of potassium too. If cells are depleted of potassium, pathological change occurs with damaging metabolic acids being produced and the cell is on its way to disease and even death. Furthermore a lack of potassium inside a cell causes sodium to fill in the vacuum and sodium increases the metabolic acidity, further causing degenerative disease and cell death. A real double-whammy.

Perky potassium can be found in (approximately in milligrams):

Lentils (100 gms)	1400
Potato, baked with skin (medium)	1250
Broad beans and peas (100 gms)	1200
Muesli, homemade (100gms)	1000
Potatoes (250 gms)	800
Nuts (100 gms)	700
Banana (medium)	450

Fish, fresh (100 gms)	450*
Vegetables, green leaf (100 gms)	350
Meat, lean organic (100 gms)	350
Orange (medium)	300
Rice, brown (100 gms)	250
Carrots (100 gms)	250
Apple (medium)	200

* Depends on the fish – can vary from 150–450

In all of the above foods, sodium levels are negligible (even in fish where it is approximately 100 mgs per 100 gms). Potassium is found in vegetables and fruit, nuts and fish, brown rice and lean organic meat (beware non-organic red meat which often has sodium salts added to it to give it better colour). Parsley and garlic, those two French staples, are also good sources.

A simple rule of thumb is also that fresh food is low in sodium and high in potassium, whilst preserved, refined and prepared foods are the opposite.

The calcium-magnesium balance

One of the biggest and worst dietary hoaxes portrayed to the Western world over the last fifty years is that osteoporosis is caused by a deficiency of calcium so we must drink more milk to correct it. This is completely inaccurate, not borne out by the scientific evidence, and just a successful end product of Milk Marketing Board PR campaigns.

People in the West have the highest levels of blood calcium in the world – thanks to dairy. And the lowest levels of bone and tissue calcium – thanks to dairy.

Let me explain. **Dodgy dairy** provides high levels of blood calcium, but this inhibits the body's uptake of zinc (crucial in helping vitamin C with its cellular and anti-cancer activities), iron (crucial for maintaining the correct oxygen levels in blood and cells), and magnesium.

The last one is significant. The daily calcium requirement for good health is just less than one gram. Amounts in excess of this will actually cause magnesium depletion.

If you inhibit the uptake of **magnificent magnesium** you cannot absorb calcium into your cellular tissues or bones. Unsurprisingly in a population awash with dairy, 2004 American research has shown that 40 per cent of adults are magnesium deficient.

Apart from magnesium, calcium also needs vitamin D to get it into the bones. Vitamin D is generated by the action of sunlight on your fat layers under the skin. Apart from this as a source, there are very small amounts in oily fish, and very, very low levels in dairy.

Magnesium is needed for vitamin D synthesis in the body. Low magnesium levels mean low vitamin D levels. So, too much dairy means high blood calcium, low magnesium and low vitamin D levels as a result. And low vitamin D levels mean low calcium absorption into bones and, worse, vitamin D deficiency is now clearly linked to a number of cancers from colon and breast cancers to brain tumours. Not surprisingly vitamin D supplementation is now being given as part of cancer therapies at a number of worldwide cancer centres.

Traditional healthy diets, from China to the Kalahari, or Greece to the Eskimos incorporate **no depressive** cow's milk. Rather, they are magnesium-rich. Magnificent magnesium-rich.

Best foods for magnesium are nuts, pulses, melons, mango, fresh sweetcorn, jacket potato, bananas, green leaves, whole grains like millet, oats, buckwheat or wheatgerm and brown rice – a similar list to that of potassium.

If you cut all dairy from your diet this instant, you could still get your daily calcium requirement from 150 gms of spinach, or from a few almonds, or any of green beans, broccoli, leeks and an orange; or dried apricots, whole grains and wheatgerm. It's really quite easy to get your daily dose of calcium. Ordinary folk in South East Asia and China don't touch dairy – and they have no osteoporosis.

But this book is about cancer and diets – importantly in the context of cancer, magnesium is also crucial to your cells because it works a little pump which sits in your cell membranes. This pump actually pumps sodium out of the cell and potassium in. Without it, sodium drifts back in to poison the cells, whilst potassium drifts out.

Magnesium is also crucial in the efficient working of your mitochondrial power stations. It prepares the fuel for burning. Without it – for example, if you are on a slimming diet – you might have terrible cravings for food when in reality you have ingested more than enough calories. Without magnesium to prepare the food you ingested and turn it into the right sort of fuel, your cells will go hungry.

Magnesium levels are also lowered by:

- Refining our foods – which removes magnesium from the grain.
- Stress and excess physical activity – which burns up magnesium in the energetic process.
- Tea, coffee, alcohol – which 'wash' magnesium out of the body.
- High sugar, carbohydrate and fat diets – which are nutritionally empty yet require magnesium for energy production.

It is not recommended that you supplement long term with magnesium. And calcium supplements that are neither organic, nor combined with magnesium can cause more harm than good. The answer is good nourishing foods – like those listed above.

Finally, magnificent magnesium is crucial to a healthy liver; a healthy liver is your crucial organ of detoxification for the whole body, and the neutraliser of nasty free radicals. Having a healthy liver is vital if you want a healthy body.

Atomic Man?

So, by eating potassium and magnesium-rich foods and limiting your intake of sodium and calcium, you will see that you have the power to change your atoms and your molecules, and with it your energy production, your body energy and even the electrical forces in and around your body?

You are indeed Atomic, and Bionic, Man (or Woman!).

CHAPTER 4
HEALTHY LIVER – HEALTHY BODY

In the UK and America few of us pay any attention to our livers. We know we have one but we don't know too much about it. Worse, we mistreat it. Day in day out.

Yet the people of China or Italy look to their livers at the first sign of illness. The routine health check I had in Beijing consists of a doctor looking into your ears and eyes, and then at your tongue. The state of the tongue will tell you much about the state of your intestines and liver; the colour of your eyes will tell you the levels of toxins present.

In France and Italy the feeling of being a bit 'rundown' is normally met with a shrug and the explanation 'une crise de foie' – a crisis of the liver. A little too much alcohol perhaps; even something they ate; and occasionally a bit of an infection. The locals will avoid fat for a few days and eat more vegetables like artichokes, fruits like melon and drink water. Why, they even have bottled waters that are well suited to reviving a flagging liver! The brand Hepar in France is magnesium rich and sells itself on its benefit to your liver.

By contrast, I cannot remember the last time a doctor in the UK looked at my tongue, nor the last time someone said they were feeling 'a bit livery'. Whatever happened to Andrews Liver Salts?

But your life depends on your liver. It is the largest organ in your body and a very complex one at that. It has a great many important functions, none more so than its ability to **detoxify the blood**: A healthy liver filters almost two pints of blood per minute, cleaning your system, so it can re-circulate and draw in more toxins and waste that your cells need to excrete.

The modern world subjects a liver to a huge range of 'poisons' which impair its function: Alcohol, pesticides, chemicals, antibiotics, drugs and external hormones like animal hormones, HRT and the contraceptive pill. Any and all of these poisons can damage the Kupffer cells, which are responsible for breaking down toxic matter, impairing the biochemical pathways and

35

reducing the performance of the liver significantly. Oestrogen can be a particularly debilitating agent, preventing the liver from detoxifying fats and generally reducing its effectiveness.

The liver also **helps make some vitamins and hormones** – it plays a role in converting precursors into vitamin D, for example.

It helps in **'energy' control systems,** being involved in providing the correct fuel for your cells from the stores of sugar and carbohydrate.

A healthy liver plays **an important role in the immune system** being involved with the white cells and even manufacturing substances like anti-histamines essential to the immune system.

One of the main jobs of a healthy liver is to **produce bile** – about three pints per day. The bile, along with its metabolic agents, the bile salts, works with the liver to metabolise fats and cholesterol and excrete waste. The process involves vast numbers of small bile ducts running throughout the liver and collecting into one common bile duct, which passes directly into the intestine. About half way along this duct sits a balloon-like object, the gall bladder, whose contractions help force the bile, along with its waste products, into the intestine.

A healthy liver also **aids digestion and absorption.** If the bile system is blocked and working inefficiently, the body's system for absorbing vitamins and minerals will be impaired. The bile works alongside enzymes, helpful bacteria and acids in the intestine to break down foods into absorbable parts. Afterwards, up to 95 per cent of the bile acids are normally reabsorbed and carried back to the liver.

Fatty livers

A fatty liver affects more than 50 per cent of adult Americans. Their carbohydrate and fat-rich diets cause a log-jam in the liver.

This is not helped by the increasing number of toxins we 'ingest'. When the liver is damaged by such toxins, it loses its efficiency to clear fats and toxins from the body, and is more likely to become 'clogged up'. If it then cannot process the fats, they will build up in the blood stream and fatty deposits will occur all over the body causing all sorts of health problems. Worse, fat is an excellent solvent and so those fatty deposits will be toxin charged, keeping free radicals, hormones and toxins in various parts of the body and creating the environment for a cancer to form.

Gallstones

Gallstones resemble small grains of sand. They are formed by cholesterol and fat collecting around clumps of bacteria, or even pieces of dead parasite (rather like a pearl forms around sand particles).

You might have none, but it is unlikely. Research showed that some 70 per cent of Americans have gallstones. Because each tends to be very small you may have as many as 3000.

Gallstones multiply the problems of fatty livers by blocking the bile ducts of the liver and preventing the free flow of the unwanted fats, cholesterol and toxins into the intestines.

However, another research study in the US showed that 99.95 per cent of cancer patients in American hospitals had gallstones, which is especially interesting as there is a school of thought that argues that every cancer patient is afflicted by microbe infection – bacteria, yeasts, parasites or virus.

Parasites abound and are on the increase. There was a four-fold increase in fluke in British livestock between 1997 and 2003, according to government figures. But parasites do not have to be large. Microscopic parasites immune to chlorine, can be carried in water systems; others on exotic vegetables and fruit. Parasites damage the liver and produce toxins like aflatoxin B, which has been linked to cancer.

The liver and cancer

If the liver function is impaired, if it is over-worked or full of fats, or blocked by gallstones, or poisoned by toxins, the whole body becomes less efficient, from the immune system to the removal of toxins from inside your cells.

It's a chain reaction. Your power stations become toxic and they pass the waste into the cell. From there it passes to the lymph and from there into the blood. Finally the wastes circulate to the liver, are 'treated' and pass into the bile, and from there out into the intestine. Block one step and the toxins find it hard to leave the power stations – the control centre for cancer.

Because the liver is involved in so many functions, there are other repercussions:

- For example, one involving the impairment of the white immune cells to recognise, attack, ingest and then bring the cancer cells for treatment in the liver.
- Or another, which involves the impairment of the body's fuel storage system resulting in lowered levels of stored fuel (glycogen) whilst increasing the fuel loved by cancer cells (glucose).

Cancer cells burn glucose, fat and protein in the absence of oxygen.

The end product of this energy production is lactic acid, in itself highly toxic. The only place lactic acid can be detoxified is in the liver and that further increases the workload.

Then, of course, the doctors give you chemotherapy drugs – and the dead cells and the toxins in the drugs will all demand processing space from the liver cells. Radiotherapy, anaesthetics, antibiotics, steroids. Let's load it up and see where the breaking point is!

What steps can we take?

We will take the extreme case, namely that of a cancer patient. People wishing to prevent a cancer can decide for themselves how much of this is relevant to their circumstances.

The start point is can you do things to flush out your liver – and other things to strengthen it.

The good news is that liver cells re-grow. Where a liver has been cut away, it will regenerate itself. Liver cells can completely detoxify themselves given the right conditions in about 8-12 weeks.

So here goes.

Cleaning out your liver

Some of you may have heard about the Gerson Therapy. It has its fans, and it has its critics. One part of it is the use of coffee enemas. Some oncology experts when criticising the Gerson

Therapy in the National Press exposed their ignorance by saying daft things like 'How can anybody expect coffee to cure cancer?' Well Gerson didn't! He used coffee enemas simply because they dilate the bile ducts and help the excretion of more of the waste – especially if there are blockages in the bile ducts. Five freshly prepared coffee enemas per day were in his original therapy, although other therapists have now reduced it to two, saying that preparing them can take a lot of time.

Another option is to use a proper liver flush. An effective liver flush and gallstone remedy is included in the Appendix. This uses a mixture of Epsom Salts, olive oil and fruit juice to clear out the blockages. You mix the Epsom Salts, olive oil and a fruit juice of your own choosing (to make the whole thing palatable) then drink a quarter at 10.00pm, another quarter at 10.30pm. Then you retire for the night. The last two quarters are consumed upon waking, and half an hour later. The effects (!) may last for two days, but people who have used it said it was all over by lunch time. One lady complained that she had excreted masses of small yellowy-green 'bits'. Well that's the bile covered gallstones. It worked. The general response amongst all users who tried it has been excellent with talk of more energy and a better feeling of health afterwards.

The simplest version – although possibly not as effective – is to take a dose of Epsom Salts once a month. A tablespoon of Epsom Salts dissolved in lukewarm water tastes foul, but the next morning after a visit to the toilet, you may well have a much cleaner liver.

Strengthening your liver

Epsom Salts contain magnesium sulphate and so provide much needed magnesium. This will help strengthen the liver (remembering that alcohol and caffeine both cause the liver stress and deplete magnesium levels). You should also major on magnesium rich foods.

Probably the best herbs are milk thistle and dandelion, which strengthen the liver system and cells. Both are better taken as liquid than pills.

Boldo tea strengthens the bile system as does globe artichoke, both promoting the excretion of fatty bile. Beets and radishes also get the juices going, as do green salads, green vegetables, spirulina, chlorella, wheat grass and barley grass.

Stopping the problem in the first place

Cutting fat out of the diet is, of course, one of the key principles seen in a number of anti-cancer diets. But it's not as simple as that. Some fats are bad – from animal fats to 'trans' fats, while some fats are good, like those in olive oil and walnut oil. Even the infamous cholesterol is recognised to have two forms now – a bad and a good.

Diets high in saturated fats, polyunsaturated fat and even refined carbohydrates should be avoided as all cause the liver to produce triglycerides. A number of research studies have shown that the cholesterol molecule is too big to get across the gut wall, and is actually re-formed on the other side. The components don't have to come from fats. They can just as easily come from carbohydrate too. So carbohydrate can just as easily give rise to your fatty liver problem.

The key issues are stopping the formation of bad fats in the body and reducing fat levels in the blood.

Perhaps the most important research finding has been on the role and involvement of beneficial bacteria in the gut. Beneficial bacteria, which are in reduced numbers in the modern body especially if you are taking prescription drugs, can break certain foods down to form short chain esters. In the blood stream these act to stop bad fats and cholesterol re-forming. We will look at beneficial bacteria in more detail later, but having enough of them in total, and enough of the right strains are a vital part of your good health, and the fight against cancer.

A diet high in lignans (plant fibre) provides factors that can bind to fats in the blood stream and help expel them from the body. The antioxidant lycopene can also do that. Lycopene is commonly found in tomatoes, tomatoes and especially cooked tomatoes.

Free radicals can literally provide the spark igniting triglycerides in the liver to become dangerous and aggressive. Vitamin E and selenium work in the liver to neutralise these free radicals. Turmeric and the B vitamins, especially choline and inositol (found in soya lecithin), will also keep them in check.

Finally, most people live in blind ignorance of the fact that they may well have a parasite. This does not have to be ten feet long. It can be microscopic – a virus, yeast, microbe or a bacterium. Up to 70 per cent of people in the Western World have excessive yeast infections (typical signs are thrush, cystitis, yellow toe nails, bloating). We will deal with this in detail in a later section.

Suffice it to say here that parasites may occupy the liver, or at minimum produce toxins and even carcinogens the liver has to deal with and which debilitate the immune system. Herbal parasite purges do exist and are usually a mixture of wormwood, slippery elm, Pau D'Arco, black walnut, clove and garlic, plus a number of immune system boosters. Interestingly Pau D'Arco was originally thought to be a 'cure' for cancer until its true action as a yeast and parasite killer was discovered. Wormwood has been found to kill yeasts and parasites but also to have a direct effect on cancer cells (Professor Lai, University of Washington). Wormwood also debilitates certain enzymes which help accumulate the high iron levels needed in cancer cells.

The final word

Love your liver!

Ignore it at your peril.

Help it, strengthen it, clean it and stop the potential problems at source.

Your diet should be its FRIEND.

CHAPTER 5
CANCER – A WEIGHTY PROBLEM

A bigger health risk than smoking

It may surprise you to know that, according to the statistics, **being obese is a bigger cancer risk factor than smoking.** I could quote you any number of studies but, by and large, smoking increases your risks of cancer by about 25 per cent and being overweight increases your risks by between 40 and 60 per cent depending on how overweight you are.

Erasmus College Rotterdam re-analysed American population data taken over a fifty-year period and concluded if you were forty years old and just four kilograms overweight you reduced your life expectancy by 3 years. At ten or more kilograms the loss was 7 years for women and 5.6 for men.

If you are ten or more kilograms overweight and you smoke, **you chop 13 years off your life expectancy.**

Be clear. 7 kgs is not a big number. I receive Personal Prescription forms from women with breast cancer who, at 5 feet 2 inches and 73 kgs, describe themselves as 'a bit chunky'. They should be around 52 kgs.

Furthermore, overweight people pay 12 per cent more visits to the doctor each year and spend 19 per cent longer per year in hospital (Men's Health UK, 2002).

Being overweight has been linked to several cancers like breast, prostate and ovarian cancer. The UK Under Secretary for Health, Hazel Blears, said, *"There are clear links between obesity and our biggest killers – heart disease and cancer."*

We have covered a number of research studies in **icon** on the links between being overweight and cancer risk. Cancer Epidemiology (Feb 13 2004) contained a study showing that women who increased weight after the age of 18 increased breast cancer risk. Over 9 kgs and risk goes up by 40 per cent, over 30 kgs and the risks double. The Fred Hutchinson Center in Seattle has directly linked obesity in women with a 20 per cent increase in breast cancer risk – they have yet to look at other cancers.

43

All is not lost though. North Carolina University has produced a study showing that women who lose their excess weight, even after developing cancer, greatly improve their survival rates.

It might be in your genes

Researchers from 77 Institutions in six countries have been analysing the DNA of 90,000 individuals. One in 17 Britons has a genetic flaw and this compounds the effects of the FTO gene discovered in 2007 to cause some people a problem in losing weight. Adults with the flaw are around three and a half pounds heavier and 24 per cent more likely to be obese than those without the flaw. However, since genes come in pairs, those people with a pair of flawed genes and two flawed copies of FTO tend to be more than 7 pounds (3.5 kgs) heavier than those 'flaw-free;. And so, according to lead researcher Dr Innes Barroso, some people will find it harder to lose weight than others.

I haven't got any answers for this – I just thought you should know! Being overweight is not always something that is your fault.

The overall problem's getting worse

The Organisation for Economic Co-operation and Development published a report in October 2002 stating that the UK has the second highest level of obesity in the world after the USA. With 21 per cent obesity we follow the USA at 26 per cent. By contrast the Swiss are Europe's best at only 6.8 per cent and the Japanese have a lowly 2.9 per cent.

One third of UK boys under six are overweight or obese, rising to almost 50 per cent by the age of 16. In the USA it is 60 per cent. The picture is worsening.

The European Conference on Oncology in 2005 heard that the UK leads Europe: 25 per cent of England's 13-17 year olds are obese. Next come Greece, Cyprus, Italy and Ireland at 23 per cent, but Germany has only 11 per cent and Holland just 9.

Puppy fat is almost a myth now. More than a quarter of schoolchildren are overweight or obese by the age of 11. Worse are girls (29 per cent) and especially black girls (38 per cent). The figure then hardly decreases at all as they age, according to CRUK.

Another study that year showed that the top ten foods of our teenagers are:

Boys	Girls
1 – Pizza	1 – Chocolate
2 – Chocolate	2 – Strawberries
3 – Ice Cream	3 – Fruit Juice
4 – Chocolate Biscuits	4 – Pasta
5 – Fruit Juice	5 – Pizza
6 – Ice Lollies	6 – Ice Cream
7 – Fizzy Drinks	7 – Grapes
8 – Pasta	8 – Ice Lollies
9 – Cakes	9 – Chocolate Biscuits
10 – Crisps	10 – Cakes

Girls eat fruit and vegetables more than boys but the average young person's diet is salt and sugar rich, biased towards refined, non-nourishing foods and, not surprisingly, they are already deficient in important minerals like magnesium, and consume virtually no 'greens' which provide essential anti-cancer vitamins like vitamin K.

47 per cent of children eat no vegetables other than potato in a month and a recent survey showed that half of ten-year-olds could not even recognise certain vegetables like broccoli correctly.

Junk food is so named for a reason. For example, only this year has McDonalds in the USA finally agreed to cut out trans fats – next year. Despite having been taken to court twice. Kellogg's is under fire in the USA. 98 per cent of their products advertised on TV have ingredients including, by weight, 35 per cent added sugars.

Several studies in 2007 have put fizzy soft drinks in the spotlight. Apart from large quantities of empty sugar, or debatable sweeteners like aspartame, there are increasing concerns over the ingredient E211 (sodium benzoate) which messes up your mitochondria, and scientists say safety limits have been set too high. Then other colourings have been linked with tissue inflammation, and a study from Harvard on 6,000 middle aged men and women showed those who drank at least one can a day were 30 or more per cent likely to be obese, have higher blood tri-glycerides and bad cholesterol.

Sadly, the UK is top of the table for the consumption of junk food in Europe with both our 5-9 and 10-13 age groups consuming more confectionary and fizzy soft drinks. Our next-to-useless Foods Standards Agency merely says this could be a warning that they will be the first generation to live shorter lives than their parents.

So, what's the problem with being overweight?

The problem with being overweight is that it has a number of consequences. For example:

- Fat is a wonderful solvent – and so stores toxins, excess hormones you would rather have excreted.
- Your hormones are more likely to be out of balance.
- Your sugar control and energy production systems are weaker.
- The excess weight puts stresses and strains on key organs, like your thyroid, pancreas and liver.

Being overweight is also indicative of other 'lifestyle' features:

- A poor diet, higher consumption of poor foods, higher toxicity, nutritional deficiency.
- A lack of sufficient exercise, a sedentary lifestyle, lowered lymph movement, lowered blood oxygen levels.
- A lack of self esteem, inattention towards one's own importance and health.

Being overweight is invariably simply due to an intake of too many calories, and the use of too few. Not only do most overweight people eat too much – they eat badly. And it causes a number of health problems and is linked to diseases like heart disease and diabetes, not just cancer.

The junk diets of the British (when compared, say to the Mediterranean Europeans) make Britons a sick bunch of people. According to a 2006 epidemiology study by Leicester University, the populations of seven out of eleven countries in Europe live longer than us – their women by up to three years more. However, we don't just die younger, we are ill longer. Apparently our women have 60.9 healthy years compared to, say, Italian women at 74.4, Spanish at 70.2 and the EU average at 66.0. Our men fair slightly better at 61.5 healthy years, compared to Italian Men at 70.9, Spanish men at 66.8 and an EU average of 64.5 years. The Mediterranean diet, sunshine, attitude to life and happiness were suggested as factors.

Moving further afield, the Okinawans have the highest life expectancy in the World, followed close behind by the Bush people. Two factors are significant. Firstly, unlike Western adults, both have reducing blood pressure as they age, probably due to the lack of sodium salt in their diets. Secondly, they have calorie restricted diets – the Okinawans consume about 40 per cent less calories than even the Japanese.

Calorie restriction

This is not the first time calorie restriction has been noted as a benefit to life expectancy. The Norwegians had their food supplies dramatically reduced by the occupying German Military during the Second World War, yet their restricted diets of fish and lowered calories resulted in a 35 per cent overall health improvement.

Research studies with rats show that calorie deprivation results in increased longevity: A 10-30 per cent reduction can almost double their life span. Harvard Researchers (**icon** 2 – 2007) have even released a video explaining how cutting the food intake of any organism by 30-40 per cent can increase longevity.

Calorie restriction has a number of benefits:

- The end benefit is that the body is slimmer and leaner. Less fat means less stored toxins.
- Calorie restriction reduces metabolic rate. Your power stations are not required to work as hard or burn as much fuel, so less waste products, toxins and free radicals are produced.
- Calorie restriction reduces insulin production, IGF-1 production, and as we will see later, this reduces the risks of both diabetes and cancer.

- The important 'added discovery' is that it increases the body's stress response – increasing survival hormones and, along with this, the body's ability to repair DNA and heighten cellular efficiency.

One hormone group vital to this process has been identified as 'sirtuins'. Whilst pharmaceutical companies are working on drugs to stimulate their production, your eat-to-beat cancer strategy can be improved by the knowledge that sirtuins are stimulated by resveratrol, a natural compound found especially in the skins of organic red grapes. It is found in all red grape, raspberry, blueberry and blackberry skins, its primary role being to stop moulds entering the fruit. Unfortunately, the use of pesticides kills the mould and less resveratrol is produced in non-organic fruits, as there is less 'mould attack'.

Not surprisingly, there are also scientific studies that show a restriction of calories can stop tumour growth.

So where do you start if you are overweight?

Most people think losing weight means starving yourself and joining a gym. Try some simple things first:

- Only buy the foods listed in the shopping list part of this book. Eating the right foods is far better than eating no foods!
- Eat a plate of salad vegetables as a starter 30 minutes before your main dinner or lunch. It will reduce the levels of 'hunger hormones'.
- Eat 6 small meals a day, not one or two big ones.
- Don't have carbohydrate and protein on the same plate – it confuses the stomach systems as we will see later, and increases fat stores. Don't eat less than two hours before going to bed.
- Yes, and try to take daily exercise. For example, walk briskly for at least 20 minutes every day (or take other forms of exercise, including stretching).
- Be proud of your body. Take care of it. It needs to last you a lifetime.

CHAPTER 6

A DIET FOR PREVENTION?

"There is a convincing body of information that proves that there is a strong dietary basis to the development of cancer."
(Jonathan Waxman, Professor of Oncology, Imperial College, London, writing in BMJ 25 November 2006)

The World Health Organisation has said as much too, concluding that 30-50 per cent of cancers are caused by 'Poor Diet', depending upon which report you read. So poor diet is one of the main 'causes', and good diet prevents.

So, what is a 'Good Diet' in the context of cancer prevention?

As this book develops you will increasingly realise that diets can, and do, help a great many people beat cancer, whether they have it already, or simply want to prevent developing it in the first place.

But is a good anti-cancer diet the UK Government's mantra of, *'A little bit of everything, based on starchy foods and 5 lots of fruit and vegetables a day'*, or is it something else?

Possible diet contenders for the Annual Cancer Prevention award include:

- The Vegetarian Diet
- The South East Asian Diet
- The Macrobiotic Diet
- The Mediterranean Diet

Adding to the confusion

There seems little doubt in some people's minds that some diets, like the Vegetarian Diet or the South East Asian Diet, are associated with lower levels of cancer. They seem excellent 'preventative' diets.

Of course 'diet' is, in itself, a terribly ambiguous word. To the great majority of women, say the word diet and they will answer,

"Which one?", or "Oh, no!" Diet to them is a wearing experience, synonymous with cutting certain, often enjoyable, foods out of their normal daily lives. The French word for diet is 'Regime', implying strictness as much as deprivation. Many health books will point you immediately in the direction of cutting out meat, and maybe dairy products, and maybe even fish too.

Obviously I know that the Vegetarian Diet involves eating no meat. But people also tell me that's the basis of the South East Asian Diet too, and I know that's not true. I live there.

Is meat eating wrong?

Yes, there is clear research that eating too much red meat increases cancer risk. Too much meat and especially saturated animal fats can increase free radicals in the body. But, too much protein *per se* can increase risks of cancer (Tannenbaum) by increasing free radicals, causing cellular changes, making your cells and your body too acid and more. (Remember, of course, that meat is not the only protein source in your diet).

Furthermore, the meat comes with the animal's own hormones, perhaps injected hormones, toxins and pesticides from the fields, and even colourings to make it look good in the shops. It's a good idea to cut it out, isn't it?

The Oxford Study on vegetarians and their diets concluded that they had 40 per cent less cancer than equivalent meat eaters. However, other information has to be factored in, for example: What if I told you that vegetarians are 80 per cent less likely to smoke? Or 60 per cent less likely to drink excess alcohol? For all I know, their increased interest in health might make them more likely to take daily exercise too. They are certainly 40 per cent less likely to be obese. To what degree does all this contribute to their 40 per cent reduced risk of cancer? Clearly diet is merely a part of their whole 'healthier lifestyle' and it is this which gives them 40 per cent less cancers. How can anyone categorically tell us that their lowered risk of cancer is totally due to eating **no** meat or animal fat?

Please believe me I'm not trying to be facetious here. I have received a couple of letters from indignant vegetarians saying that all the evidence points to a meat-free diet being highly protective. But what evidence? To be sure you would need matched samples of people with identical lifestyles and diets save for the meat and animal fat and dairy eating.

I am also concerned about the real possibility of cancer resulting from vitamin and mineral deficiencies. For example a little over 60 per cent of breast cancer patients seem to have vitamin B-12 deficiency. A Vegetarian Diet could make matters worse. Three quarters of vegetarians are known to be deficient in B-12, as the prime source is meat. (So, if you do decide to become vegetarian after cancer is diagnosed, please take chlorella, an excellent natural source of minerals, enzymes and certain vitamins – like vitamin B-12 and beta-carotene).

Sally Beare in her book *The Live Longer Diet* studied longevity in various populations, and the Okinawans and the Bush People come top. The former eat fresh fish, the latter a little wild meat, and they both live longer than vegetarians. Vegetarians also don't actually live longer than an equivalent sample of health conscious, meat eating, non-smokers either. One important reason is that they still eat salt and sugar and these are important factors in restricting life-span.

One man's meat

Moreover, one man's meat can really be another's poison. Peter D'Adamo has written a very good book on choosing the right foods for your blood type: *Eat Right for Your Type*. In this book, he tracks how populations moved out of Africa and developed different blood types around the world. These different types actually thrive on different foods, often the foods that surrounded them over many thousands of years. The fittest adapt and grow stronger in tune with their localised, natural environments.

Choosing what is best for you and your personal biochemistry is called 'Metabolic Typing'. It has been taken to a fine art form by experts like Bill Wallcott in the USA who use blood tests or hair samples and can tell you that some people have a body biochemistry that thrives on meat eating, while others would do better to avoid it.

So, while I acknowledge that eating meat and animal fats can be an increased risk factor for some people, I am actually more interested in trying to learn what foods we should be building into our diets to try to beat cancer.

The South East Asian Diet

Frankly, a lot of rubbish is talked about the South East Asian Diet, mostly from people who have never been near the place and merely pass on their interpretation of other people's interpretation of someone who visited once. I will try to give you an accurate feeling for the real South East Asian Diet.

I have travelled extensively in the region, from Vietnam, to Cambodia to rural China. I live in Thailand and my wife is Khmer – a vast area that crosses from East Thailand, through Laos and Cambodia. Cancer is almost non-existent and, personally although I do think that their diet is part of the reason, I think other factors are actually more important.

The Khmer eat soup for breakfast – made from boiling rice with herbs, chopped spring onions, garlic and ginger (or galangal), and a little chicken, pork or fish. Lunch is also soup – possibly the dish known as Tom Yum Kung in the West, a boiled river prawn or fish dish with herbs, galangal, lemon grass, tomatoes and a little coconut milk. Alternatively, if they are out working in the fields, they will take sticky rice with them in little circular 'hampers' plus bits of fish and slices of green mango. Dinner might be 'barbequed' chicken, duck or river fish with vegetables, or Som Tam, a salad styled dish consisting of shredded green mango, papaya, cucumber, green beans, onions, tomato, herbs and carrot all mixed in a fish sauce with lime juice, chilli and garlic – very spicy. They might even throw in a river prawn or a small river crab.

Only in towns and cities is food fried in woks. In the rural areas it is boiled, or they grill it or bake it in improvised ovens. They never add salt – but do have thyroid problems from a lack of iodine, and sea salt is now extensively farmed along the coast.

They nibble at vegetables and fruit all day – they seem to be eating all the time. Fruit, which is fresh and sweet, is everywhere. Mangoustein, lychees, papaya, bamboo shoots, watermelon, rambutan, durian, pommello, bananas, pineapple and many more. When Thais come to Europe they complain that our fruit is sour – and it is, because it has been picked unripe to travel and then last longer in our supermarkets.

They eat a lot of chilli (mainly in the evenings) and garlic and spring onions. Frankly, a lot of their vegetables resemble bits of twig and grass, but are fragrant so I guess are more correctly termed herbs.

Chickens run wild everywhere; they do have ducks, pigs and lots of cows and water buffalo, which they eat immediately after killing them; and they fish the rivers and lakes continuously. So you can see straight away that it is a fallacy that they are vegetarian, or too poor to eat meat. A home can have 5 cows, 3 water buffalo and sixty chickens. In China the markets are full of chickens and pork meat. Oh, and dead field rats and gutted, skinned dogs. In the North of Thailand and in Laos and China they eat certain wild birds, snails, whole frogs – not just the legs – and fried beetles and cockroach-like flies. They eat lots of eggs and even snakes.

They do not touch milk, and only recently has soya and sweetcorn milk come in packs to their villages. Interestingly the soya milk is 'reinforced with milk protein' according to the pack.

But, their food has no pesticides. They are scrupulously clean, but they use no make up or perfumes or toiletries. Their stone floors are swept clean and household cleaners and bleach unheard of.

Their natural exercise levels are high. One report about the Chinese showed that their natural exercise consumes 3,600 calories per week. You would need to go to the gym and work out for one hour per day to equal this. They walk everywhere (in China they cycle!), they make everything themselves – houses, furniture, fences etc and they are fit. My wife's father at seventy years of age is solid muscle, the sort of physique you see on the front cover of 'Men's Health'.

They go to bed at eight-thirty at night (it gets dark at six-thirty) and sleep in total darkness. They wake at first light, and get up.

They smoke little, but drink in excess: Beer (every region has its own brand), rice wine and 'whisky' (which is really rum, because it is made from sugar).

They have two or three children – bribery helps get round the rules in China – and wouldn't dream of not breast feeding them for about 9 months.

Their life expectancy, in my opinion, is lower than ours because they work so hard, outdoors in the sun and they simply get tired. It is also an issue of statistics – they have greater infant mortality and that reduces the average age of death, compared to the West. However, given that 80 per cent of cancers occur in the over 65 age group in the West, you can also see how many of them might not even be living long enough to develop the disease!

They are the happiest people I have ever come across – any excuse and they are dancing and laughing, being poor is just 'bad luck'. If someone is rich, it is their 'good luck', so jealousy is unheard of. If you have good luck then you share it with your family and friends. And the monks. And then you will come back in the next life luckier still.

Everyone eats 'a bit of dirt' daily. Hands touch cows or dogs and pass bits of chicken to you to eat, or scoop sticky rice up for the children's mouths.

Overall, the cancer rate in Thailand (which has the same population as the UK), is a quarter of ours. But, 'rich persons' disease' is growing. The Thai Health Minister has already been on the front page of the national newspapers urging Thais to get back to their historic diets and telling them to avoid the American fast food outlets. He'd be sued if he said that in Britain.

Burger King, McDonalds, Starbucks, and various pizza parlours have arrived. So too has Tesco with its household cleaners and arrays of perfumes and soaps. And also mobile phones and masts, and even WiFi in the towns' hotels. Doctors now dish out antibiotics for everything. Toyota now have a showroom in the village. And there is even talk of GM crops. No doubt they'll soon be offered mortgages!

So, please don't be confused. In my opinion, yes, their diets are a contributory factor to their low cancer rates – starting with no frying, the consumption of lots of vegetables and fruit and lean wild meat and fish, but also no salt and no dairy. Lemon grass, galangal and kafir lime leaves – used frequently in their soups – are three of the most potent antioxidant-containing foods known; the active ingredient of lemon grass is almost 300 times more powerful than beta-carotene in carrots. Papaya and bamboo shoots contain good levels of vitamin B-17. But we have natural compounds in our native foods in Europe that are equally potent.

A second area of benefit is that they ingest lots of beneficial bacteria, no antibiotics and drugs, and the coconut (caprylic acid), garlic, onions and chillis kill off yeasts and microbes – their digestive systems and the blood systems work and are 'clean'. (See Chapter 23)

They sleep naturally in the dark – whereas, sleeping in artificial lighting and sleep deprivation due to night shift work are actually being declared known carcinogens by IARC – The European cancer body.

Happiness helps build a strong immune system too, as does plenty of all day exercise, and they have none of the stresses of the Western World to weaken it.

Finally, they are chemical and pesticide-free. And they are also, usually, thin

Now please tell me that I should adopt a meat-free South East Asian Diet if I want to beat cancer.

Cancer is a lifestyle disease

The important thing is to be open-minded, rational and to start to learn from this. We might conclude that eating a little wild meat and fish, no dairy, lots of vegetables and fruits can help you prevent cancer – but it's a bit woolly. And it certainly isn't much of a plan.

What I think both diets do tell us is that you really cannot separate diet from the total lifestyle. To suggest, if you want to beat cancer, that you should just bolt a new diet onto an existing, possibly flawed lifestyle is nonsense.

Cancer is 'rich person's disease' and rich people eat more, are fatter, drive around in cars, using household chemicals and personal toiletries, live on mobile phones, have more stress, sleep poorly (often with street lights outside their windows), do less manual work and so on. When Chinese people go to live in the USA they adopt the US illness rates and cancer statistics very quickly. Cancer is a lifestyle disease.

And if you develop cancer **you need to mend your whole life –** the full width of it. Diet is just one aspect.

CHAPTER 7
MENDING A LIFE

In balance with your environment

One's environment, one's lifestyle, one's diet and one's health are all interlinked, as is one's soul and one's mental attitude to the community at large and the greater universe. A disease in an individual is an affliction on the community, a measure of its failings, and cannot be thought of as separate or confined to the individual.

Is this a crank view? I suggest you read the paragraph slowly and carefully again.

Giraffes have long necks because the ones with short necks couldn't reach the leaves on the trees and died out. Over hundreds of thousands of years these leaves best nourished the giraffes' biochemistry and the biochemistry was built on that nourishment. So too papaya best nourishes someone in the Philippines, an apple someone in Austria, whale meat best nourishes an Eskimo and oats a Scotsman.

But it is not just food that nourishes the biochemistry. Buddhism nourishes the body in Bhutan, yoga in Lahore. Praise might nourish a child in Paris; criticism might depress a cleaner in Cologne.

Naturopathy is an ancient system of healing, which encourages building your immunity naturally by viewing the individual as an integral part of nature's big picture.

Conventional medicine and naturopathy overlap in the study of Psycho-Neuro-Endocrino-Immunology or PNEI. Put simply: Our feelings, emotions and thoughts are fundamentally connected through the nervous, energy and hormone systems to all the workings of our bodies.

And it is easy to see how lifestyle, food and diet can affect the lot – and quite quickly. For example:

- Stress greatly increases your cortisol levels. Doctors normally send patients home to rest for a week. Seattle Medical Centre showed us, in matched research samples, that your first ever yoga lesson can reduce cortisol levels by 25 per cent compared with just a 5 per cent drop after a full week in the stay-homers.

- Meditation causes changes in the hypothalamus, which through the pituitary gland affects the whole body. The New York Presbyterian Hospital has shown us in clinical trials that meditation before surgery can reduce blood loss by 40 per cent.
- Several universities have shown us that depression is related to lower blood oxygen levels. Pennsylvania and UCLA have shown that blood oxygen levels can be raised through exercise. And this can relieve depression.
- Aggressive children can find themselves locked up in state institutions in the USA if their aggression has lead to crime. Several research studies have shown that supplementation with fish oils (omega-3) considerably alters the levels of aggression, through changes to the brain biochemistry

So, just as our diets affect our biochemistry, so our stresses, our depressions, our aggressions can affect it – they are all inter-linked.

Of course, some mental states are caused by diet – alcohol would be the most obvious example, but too much, or too little sugar can also cause dramatic effects in some people. Then there are illnesses due to deficiencies or sensitivities. We all understand that we may have food intolerances. Some are extreme: I have a friend who cannot eat shell fish – he goes bright red, can't breathe and has to be rushed to hospital.

Physical factors, mental factors, diet, lifestyle, our historical, local surrounding and the nourishment they provided. They are all inter-woven.

The Macrobiotic Diet

Between 1896 and 1907 a Japanese army officer was, even then, deeply concerned at the Westernisation of the traditional Japanese diet and he implored the Japanese people to re-embrace their traditional healthy values.

Sagen Ishizuka went 'back to basics' and stated his fundamental belief that the food we eat not only sustains life, it makes for our basic health and happiness. He set up a clinic and started to treat hundreds of patients with the principles of Yin and Yang, and the traditional Japanese peasant diet. His fame and success brought him the title of the 'anti-doctor,' not because he was against doctors but because his disciples simply didn't need them!

In the 1950s George Ohsawa brought Ishizuka's diet and principles to the West. Later, Michio Kushi consolidated his work and there is a Kushi Institute in London.

And that was how **macrobiotics** started. Sadly, the use of the diet by certain media stars has caused some people to ridicule or trivialise the value of the diet. But it is simple, sensible and sound.

The term itself comes from the Greek: *macro* meaning 'great' or 'long' and *biotic* meaning, 'concerning life'. The original word was attributed to Hippocrates, the father of modern medicine. However the concept of macrobiotics is not focused on diet *per se* but rather the ancient Chinese belief that all life, indeed the whole universe, is a balance of two opposing forces Yin and Yang.

Unlike most modern-day diets, many of which give the feeling of having been created or invented often with slimming in mind, macrobiotics is best described by the phrase 'back to basics' – for your food and for you and your health.

Yin elements in the macrobiotic diet are regarded as cold, slow, filling and weak; Yang in contrast is quick, dry and hard. Most disease, and especially cancer, is regarded as having a Yin cause. However for any individual all aspects of their life should be assessed by Yin and Yang principles, not just their diet. Any excess thought to be causing an illness can then be corrected or counterbalanced by providing foods of the opposite force.

The five basic principles are that:

- Foods are the foundation of health and happiness.
- Sodium and potassium are opposites in food, reflecting opposing Yin and Yang Forces
- Man's staple food is grain.
- Food should be unrefined, whole and natural.
- Food should be grown locally, ripe and consumed in season.

If you meet with a macrobiotic consultant concerning a cancer do not be surprised if he delves into everything in your past from diet to lifestyle, from illnesses to allergies. To undertake macrobiotics is to try to mend your whole life.

He is likely to recommend a core diet, around which he will introduce specific foods particular to your needs. It should be noted that a fundamental tenet of macrobiotics is that every one of us is an individual and one man's grain is another man's poison.

The core diet is likely to include:

- Whole grains (e.g. millet, barley, brown rice).
- Vegetables (including pulses and some fruits).
- Seaweed and sea vegetables.
- Fermented soya products (e.g. tofu, shoyu and miso soup).
- Regular consumption of oily fish.
- Monounsaturated oils.
- Japanese low caffeine green tea.

Whenever possible, everything should be fresh, and freshly prepared. Freshly prepared juices may also be recommended, but raw food may not at the outset as, even if vegetables are only blanched, cooked foods supposedly have more 'fire', more energy. Dairy, sugar and meat are likely no-go foods. Organic food predominates and the diet may be extended to include exercise, yoga and even a little meditation.

A change to a macrobiotic diet and lifestyle has helped many people achieve a new health, and it has helped many cancer patients. It does require a little effort and time, but it does not have to be forever. Some people find its corrective action may only be needed for a year or so.

Some argue that the use of grains, whole or otherwise, in a modern world that stores them in silos and finds them developing moulds and carcinogenic aflatoxins, should be cut out, while others argue that this established, hundred-year-old viewpoint places too much emphasis on cooked rather than raw foods. However, I think it is an excellent starting point on our search for the best anti-cancer diet, not least because the Japanese traditionally had such small rates of cancer (pickled food, high salt consumption and smoking is changing all that).

Of course, the macrobiotic diet is not dissimilar to the diet still used by the Okinawans we refered to earlier. Surrounded by a coral sea, their diet has less carbohydrate (and therefore calories) than even the Japanese diet, and small amounts of protein from fish and vegetables. They have an extremely high organic mineral intake, the lowest cancer rates in the world bar none, and an average life expectancy of 81.2 years, the highest in the world.

Locally grown, fresh, ripe fruit and vegetables is a very sensible rule for delivering the most nourishment from your natural foods – how can picking a fruit half ripe, storing it in nitrogen, shipping it across the world, 'ripening' it in the shop window and eating it 4 weeks after it was picked be expected to bring nourishment to your body? Why, in Britain, do we want to eat lychees, rice and mangoes from China when our ancestors have built their biochemistry with nourishment from apples, pears and potatoes?

The fundamental point about macrobiotics is that it is a plan which is totally adaptable to you and your local environment wherever you live. It is flexible, but has disciplined underlying principles. The core elements are very protective and effective against cancer and the avoidance of most dairy, sugar and meat makes a contribution too. Whole grains have their vitamins, minerals and fibre content intact; pulses provide protective plant oestrogens, as does the fermented soya. Oily fish contribute small amounts of vitamins E and D, and large amounts of anti-inflammatory omega 3.

The diet is part of a new life tailored to the individual's problems and needs and my only concern would be the use of non-local foods for the average Westerner.

But it's a start. A set of principles in a plan. A plan that is about width and tackling the totality that is the illness or cancer process. Do we have a plan like this in the West?

CHAPTER 8
THE FRENCH CONNECTION

The following statements are all true:

- The Japanese eat very little fat and suffer fewer heart attacks and cancers than us.
- The Mexicans eat a lot of fat and suffer fewer heart attacks and cancers than us.
- The Chinese drink very little red wine and suffer fewer heart attacks and cancers than us.
- The Italians drink excessive amounts of red wine and suffer fewer heart attacks and cancers than us.
- The Eskimos eat more fat than anyone else in the world, and they have less heart attacks and cancers than us.
- The French eat more fat than us, and drink excessive amounts of red wine, and even they suffer fewer heart attacks and cancers than us.

Conclusion? Eat and drink what you like. Speaking English is apparently what kills you.

A low fat, high carbohydrate diet?

For thirty years or so from the mid 1960's, Western Governments and dietary experts talked about a healthy eating pyramid. Do you remember? Lots of foods at the bottom that you can eat once a year, and two or three foods at the top that you are supposed to make meals out of every day. 'High fibre' – so everyone rushed out to buy their Super Bran flakes; 'high carbohydrate' – so everyone started eating rice and pasta; 'low fat' – so everyone bought low fat spreads and low fat yoghurts.

The truth is that adding fibre as an extra to your diet does little for you – the fibre needs to be inherent in the food, wrapped around the sugar stores to ensure their slow release. High carbohydrate diets pushed people (especially women looking to slim) into meals of refined, nutritionally useless wheat pasta. And then there's low fat. How ignorant and misleading that seems nowadays.

The French Paradox

It also meant that these dietary experts had to ignore the opening little commentary at the start of this chapter. Joke or not, it is true. And for the Western World the biggest dietary lesson was simply swept under the carpet. The French diet, dubbed a paradox as if it were some paranormal, unexplainable Gallic mystery, sat uneasily with the superficial approval given to the Asian Diet or vegetarian studies.

The French paradox? The French eat more fat than the Americans and British, and consume more alcohol. Yet they have lower rates of cancer and heart diseases, they spend 30 per cent less on health care and enjoy a longer average life expectancy. Several studies have produced this same data. One actually showed that within France the area of highest fat consumption was in Gascony – the home of D'Artagnan, broad, beefy rugby playing men and their well built wives. It is also the home of foie gras, pates, sausages, many cheeses, cream and of dishes like cassoulet (pork fat, duck breast, bacon and sausages in a bean stew).

And where do the French have the least cancers and heart attacks? In Gascony.

Factors that protect

Ignoring the French Paradox was the biggest mistake dietary experts ever made – they still do it today. Because it tells us something incredibly important. The priority isn't cutting out the harmful animal fats. The priority is adding foods into your diet that can counteract – that can protect and correct.

One of my best friends lives in Gascony – spend a week or two there. It's a farming community, so plenty of beneficial bacteria in your daily diet, plenty of leeks, onions and garlic, especially chopped and raw. Salads covered in olive oil; red wine with every meal; fruits in abundance throughout the summer and autumn. (They are like the Thais, always nibbling at a fruit.) They exercise, they play rugby and they move bales of straw. And they eat. Eating is a fundamental pleasure in life – it is a national sport.

Importantly, they believe in 'nourishment' – in real food. I was talking to the local hairdresser about McDonalds. *'Why would we want one here? My children like their food'*, he said. No coincidence then that McDonalds near Ste Maxime is almost only populated by tourists, and had to provide a range of salads (including prawn, and smoked salmon) plus proper potatoes not merely French Fries, to get any French customers into the place. If a French woman wants to diet, she merely eats smaller portions – she wouldn't think of changing what she eats. The British and the American seem to have this belief that in some way you can eat yourself slim. Carry on – just switch to low calorie or low fat versions and the pounds will drop off! Who in their right mind would drink a gin and slimline tonic?

Have you seen the film 'Green Card'? There is a wonderful scene that sums a lot of this up. The mighty Gaul, Gerard Depardieu, is having breakfast with his American leading lady, Andie McDowell. Incredulous at her breakfast offerings, he goes out and buys a coffee percolator, and his full butter croissants. When she has her muesli, covered in low fat yoghurt – he looks on in disgust. *'birdseed'*, he mutters under his breath.

The Mediterranean Diet

One area of France has a diet that does pass muster with the Politically Correct Dietary Brigade and that is the Mediterranean Diet. And, yes I know it's getting boring, but I have first-hand experience of this diet too, as I've had a house in France by the Mediterranean for 23 years.

The northern Mediterranean, in a diet definition, seems to stretch only from Marseille to somewhere near Naples. The diet typically includes:

- A limited amount of meat.
- A limited amount of dairy (from goats).
- Red wine consumption with meals.
- Good consumption of fresh nuts.
- Good consumption of dried fruits.
- High consumption of vegetables, including garlic.
- High consumption of whole grains.
- High consumption of fruits.

- High consumption of olive oils and nut oils (monounsaturated oils).
- High percentage of home-grown, in season, fresh and organic produce.
- High consumption of fish.

The coast line of the Northern Mediterranean is an extended fishing community. The boats still come in every day, and serve their catch at the quayside in France and Italy. Go in land 25 kilometers and you are in farming communities.

Tomatoes, peppers, beetroot, onions, cucumbers and salads. Peaches, oranges, plums, pears, apples. Everything has its season. In May it will be asparagus and strawberries, in June it will be peaches and salad vegetables and so on through apricot season, to the Nut Festivals when the châtaigne (chestnuts) and walnuts are picked. Fresh, local, in-season produce. And they've never heard of macrobiotics!

From my local knowledge I can tell you that the locals shop at the local farms, not the supermarket. 18 per cent of the local produce is organic; they use crop rotation. Our oil is only olive oil or occasionally walnut. Olive oil is dribbled on everything. You even dip your bread in it before your meal. Grilled fish is the staple along the coast, in-land there is a lot of wild game. Of course you can have the fish stew, or the fish soup. The fishermen of Marseille invented bouillabaisse using the ugly fish in their catch that no one could sell. Salad Nicoise? It's not the one you have in London. It was made of lettuce, green beans, onions and tomatoes with the little anchovies the fishermen of Nice couldn't sell, all covered in olive oil and chopped garlic.

The standard cooked vegetable dish is ratatouille – peppers, courgettes, aubergines, onions and garlic stewed with olive oil. Nothing is fried, no salt added.

The fennel, onions and garlic kill any harmful microbes and yeasts I consume. Everything is flavoured with herbs. Thyme, marjoram, rosemary, mint and basil. Even saffron has been shown to have three anti-cancer compounds (crocin, picrocin and safranal).

Coffee is strong and black. Cheese is likely to be from goats as the hinterland is mountainous. Little cows' dairy was consumed traditionally, although the consumption of cheeses is increasing nowadays. And then of course there is the wine. And the sun on our skins which makes vitamin D in our bodies. St Tropez has 3,000 hours of sunshine a year. It's an outdoor life. Simple brick houses with stone floors to keep the heat out in summer and the cold north wind out in winter. At night you sleep in the pitch black, with shutters on the windows, an historical requirement, to protect you from thieves.

Atkins Diet? The 'No-grain diet'? The cabbage diet? What rubbish is that?

Research approves!

Fat? In 2002 a European survey concluded that people on the Mediterranean consumed the highest levels of fat, yet had the lowest levels of heart attacks and cancers in Europe.

Salt? While the UK Food Standards Agency is still stuck in a rut telling us all that adults should eat 6 gms of salt a day and children 3 gms, the Mediterranean diet incorporates less than a tenth of that amount.

And now someone has actually researched the Mediterranean diet and published a paper in the Journal of the American Medical Association. In this, two groups of people were studied comprising over 2000 men and women all aged between 70 and 90 at the start of the eleven year study. (Importantly, they did not separate food from local lifestyle.) Here are the conclusions:

- The benefits of diet, alcohol, exercise and non-smoking were described as **dramatic**. People who followed the Mediterranean lifestyle had 65 per cent less risk of death over the control group!!!
- Each of the following areas <u>independently</u> provided benefit:
  *The diet – high in fruit, vegetables, nuts, fish, olive oil, seeds and whole grains, but low in meat and meat products – cut risk of death by 23 per cent.
  * Exercise – defined as 30 minutes per day of moderate activity – cut risk of death by 37 per cent.
  * **Alcohol** – those people drinking one to four glasses of wine

per day – cut risk of death by 22 per cent. (Indeed non-drinkers were significantly worse off.)
* **Non-smoking** – not one cigarette consumed in the past 15 years – cut risk of death by 34 per cent.

And if you do all four, the total figure is 65 per cent across the eleven-year period.

In the November 2007 Edition of the FASEB Journal, French researchers have shown that the real beneficial issue with the French diet is the polyphenol content. Polyphenols are plant compounds and there are several thousand different ones. Many are powerful antioxidants and the scientists showed that they could both prevent and shut down tumours by cutting off the formation of new blood vessels needed for tumour growth. The study also showed dose dependency, with increasing effects as more and different polyphenols were consumed, and showed the benefits for people with heart and circulatory problems. The scientists, in particular, reviewed the 'Mediterranean Diet' and found the polyphenol content of fruits, vegetables, herb teas and red wine was extremely high and very potent – red wine started to have a beneficial effect at the level of just one glass!

A colourful life

The South of France is a colourful place – its regional hues are blue, orange, yellow and green.

Now imagine that every day in the centre of our big lunch table we have a one metre long concave piece of tree bark filled with vegetables – fennel, tomatoes, yellow peppers, red peppers, beetroot, cauliflower, radishes, cucumber, sweetcorn, onions, spring onions, garlic cloves. And the one for fruit with apricots, peaches, deep red plums, cherries, strawberries, grapes.

The yellows, the reds, the whites, the greens and the deep purples are all plant pigments that protect. They may be called flavenoids, or polyphenols, or carotenoids or anthocyanins but that doesn't matter to someone living in the South of France or Gascony. They are just part of life's rich tapestry. The vegetables and fruits have all drawn minerals from an ever changing soil. A soil that uses natural manure and organic farming practices. A soil much of which is continuously silted by the rivers coming down from the mountains. Foods for enjoyment; food that nourishes, protects and prevents, as does the wine, the olive oil, the fresh nuts and the sun.

To my mind any diet for health should start with the French Diet as a lesson. Whether from Gascony, where the fats are counteracted by red wine, olive oil, garlic, onions and plentiful vegetables and fruits and nuts. Or the South of France and the benefits of the natural compounds in fish soup, ratatouille, garlic, herbs, vegetables and fruits and nuts. They may smoke and eat too much and they may well be overweight. But they enjoy their outdoor life, and they live longer than we do in the UK, and with their first serious illness coming well after ours.

This would seem to be a diet that protects and corrects – a diet that nourishes and heals. And the sheer volume of fruits and vegetables provides the width to combat various aspects of the cancer process. The most telling factor in the research to my mind is the finding that this was 'dose dependent' – the more you eat – in terms of volume and width – the lower your risk of illness.

CHAPTER 9
A DIET FOR PEOPLE WITH CANCER?

Some UK professors and oncologists will tell you that if you already have a cancer, no diet is going to help you stop the cancer. In fact, one top cancer expert and professor wrote a point of view in the *British Medical Journal* about exactly this, saying he had many studies all showing that changing your diet didn't matter a jot to the outcome. (Sadly, no references for these studies were contained with the article.)

This of course is excellent news for oncologists everywhere. Firstly, it excuses their ignorance on nutrition: Hippocrates was wrong – food can never be medicine. And secondly, it will scare patients into believing that the only way they can possibly beat their cancer is to trust their oncologist and his orthodox therapies, as this complementary and alternative stuff blatantly doesn't work.

I find this sort of comment truly amazing. It is demoralising for patients at best, and, at worst, it is quite inaccurate.

So – is it worth changing your diet to beat your cancer?

Moreover, suggesting changing diet has no effect on cancer outcomes so you shouldn't bother, is actually in conflict with the UK's National Cancer Plan (2000), where part of the plan was that patients should be given nutritional advice in order to improve their outcomes! The plan ran for 5 years (I am also obliged to ask, 'So, what changed during that time?!')

Next came the 2007 report of the World Cancer Research Fund and the American Institute of Cancer Research entitled 'Food, Nutrition, Physical Activity and the Prevention of Cancer – a Global Perspective.' It was the largest ever review of research on diet and cancer, and even studied diet and cancer type. Unfortunately, the evidence was too limited to draw any conclusions on a specific diet to prevent cancer. (!)

However, waiting for this report on 'prevention' was cited as one reason for the delays in effecting the nutritional advice as per the UK's 2000 National Plan (for people who already had the disease).

Confused? Sometimes I want to cry.

One real concern I have is that many of the 'let's see if a diet really can beat cancer' studies are just naïve. Chucking a few antioxidant vitamins like E, C and beta-carotene down patient's throats, and/or seeing if they live longer if they have cut out red meat is certainly not what this book is about at all. However, I fear it is what many doctors mean by people changing their diets.

The fact is that 'Diet' is acknowledged as crucial for the prevention of cancer – and in 2000 the UK 'Cancer Powers' decided it was important to give people nutritional advice to improve their odds of survival. Diet is a crucial element for everyone who wants to beat cancer.

For example as we will see later, Nobel Prizes have been won for showing natural compounds in your diet can reduce inflammation, while others for showing how natural diet compounds can help your immune system better recognise cancer cells. Suppose your condition merits anti-oestrogen drugs (like Arimidex). Why shouldn't you help your doctor with a diet that limits oestrogen too?

Furthermore for many, many people with cancer, the doctors have told them at some point that they are 'All Clear'. If a good diet is totally accepted as a way of reducing cancer risk and preventing its occurrence, doesn't it make simple sense to employ one at this time? After all, breast cancer drugs are used in much the same way – to prevent a cancer occurring in the other breast, according to Professor Howell at our Cancer Prevention Conference. Why not also use a good diet to increase your personal odds of preventing the cancer occurring in the other breast too?

Finally, there is an important issue that many doctor's just can't get their heads round: **Self-empowerment**. Many people who have cancer simply want to take back control of their own life at this point – they do not want some doctor and his, often limited, orthodox medicine and statistics to have total control over their lives. And so over half of all patients in the UK hit the internet to find other things they can do – from changing diet to taking supplements to taking up yoga and having an Indian head massage. So called 'Quack Busters', doctors who think they know better, jump to criticise saying there is no research evidence that these things help, and where there is improvement, saying that *'It's a placebo effect'* (an effect not produced by the chemical or biochemical effect of the treatment but due to unrecognised forces from the brain – for example, a 'feel good factor'). Frankly most people with cancer don't care what causes the improvement in their health, or their side-effects. Their improvement may well be 'all in the mind'; so what? It is increasingly acknowledged anyway that the medical profession knows very little about mental state and cancer. Jumping to criticise the use of acupuncture or Indian head massage as a placebo just highlights this ignorance!

At CANCERactive we have heard too many stories of patients asking their doctors about diet improvements and diet therapies only for the doctor to tell them their efforts are worthless, and even ridiculing the patient. To these few people I offer the words of George Bernard Shaw: *"It is easy . . . terribly easy . . . to shake a man's faith in himself. To take advantage of that, to break a man's spirit, is the devil's work."*

Frankly the medical profession has only itself to blame if it has lost control of the patients. Perhaps a course in nutrition and complementary therapies so that oncologists can discuss such matters knowledgably and objectively with their patients would be a good place to start if they want to regain some respect?

Every person has the right to take control of their own lives – to mend themselves – especially when faced with cancer. Every person has a duty to themselves to employ the best Complementary and Alternative Therapies available to increase their personal odd of survival – and that includes having a great diet.

Rushing to correct

Be clear, diets have helped a great many people beat cancer. But sadly, all too many people just rush into this enormous area, sometimes at great personal deprivation giving up their favourite foods, and end up doing bits and bobs, which could never do enough to attack the whole process that is cancer in their bodies.

Many cancer patients 'rush' into a supposedly corrective diet, cutting out meat, dairy and all manner of foods and consuming multi-vitamins and some tincture the lady down the road said cured her brother. This may be due to peer group pressure, or it may simply be a desire to 'do the very best for myself' and 'to take back some control over my own body, my own health, my own life'. Such 'deprivation' diets are not 'wrong' – it's just that by the end of this book you will realise that you could be doing so much more for yourself.

Towards a dietary discipline

There is a whole heap of supposed 'Diets' for cancer patients: From Dr Ferenczi and his beetroot diet, to Joanna Brand, a South African naturopath, who cured her cancer by eating organic grapes and little else.

The problem is that helpful friends, 'alternative' health practitioners, even the Press bombard you with this week's miracle cure and wonder diet. Yes, beetroot contains anthocyanins which can kill cancer cells. And I have no reason to doubt that eating grapes probably worked for Joanna Brand and I'm extremely happy for her. However, as I've shown already, the causes of cancer are very individual and it is a multi-stage disease. And something may be wondrously successful for one person and their cancer in its stages, yet totally useless for someone else who has many more or different stages.

Unfortunately the matter doesn't end there. Sadly, some people 'cure' themselves with a diet, then open a clinic thinking they can do the same for everybody's cancer – and it simply doesn't work like this. They make sweeping, often totally subjective comments, utter generalisations without evidence, and are rightly accused of being little more than quacks. They do the genuine dietary practitioners and cancer patients a disservice because they add to the general confusion and detract from the real Diet Therapies with proven-in-research track records that do cure people.

As we have seen, it would seem that certain diets, like the Vegetarian Diet or the South East Asian Diet, may be associated with lower levels of cancer, if indeed you can separate the diet from the lifestyle. But does that make them relevant if you already have it?

I believe it is quite irresponsible of people to suggest cancer patients simply adopt these diets in the belief they might cure a cancer. As I keep saying, cancer is a disciplined multi-stage process, and it needs a disciplined multi-faceted response and I don't see too much discipline in either of these diets. As I've already suggested, cutting meat out of a cancer patients' diet might add to their problems.

I could be wrong of course. There are many Help Centres and Clinics you can use and they do believe people with cancer should give up meat eating: For example, Dr Johanna Budwig, at her clinic, uses a vegetarian/raw food diet with flaxseeds and quark, the Hippocrates Health Institute in Boston use organic wheat grass and a vegetarian diet. They may well all have built a multi-disciplined approach to the problem and be getting great results – I hope so.

In the UK, The Penny Brohn Cancer Care Centre in Bristol, (formerly the Bristol Cancer Help Centre) has actually pulled back from the brink of telling people to 'go vegetarian'. They, like me, think some people may thrive on meat and recommend a limited amount of white meat. (My view is that you can have a limited amount of meat, ideally free range or game and certainly organic.) Again, like me, they follow the very latest research and try to incorporate a width of specific foods into the diet to do a specific job. Also, like me, they see diet as a part of a wider programme of therapies, intended to rebuild your whole life.

Unfortunately, when I asked this well-respected organisation if they had numbers on their success, as of March 2008, they didn't. But I do know that they are looking into the issue.

This highlights another issue. It is all too easy for orthodox 'experts' to jump to criticise Diet Therapies because there are no hard numbers – no clinical trials. I find it very hard to imagine how there are ever going to be. Inevitably patients who follow a healthy diet route incorporate other complementary therapies into the healing programme too. How are the researchers going to get perfectly matched samples – this group had surgery, radio and chemotherapy – the other also changed their diet? And who would pay for the research – all the organic foods and supplements? The charity health clinics certainly can't afford to!

But it would be quite wrong to assume that all Diet Therapies – i.e. full disciplined programmes to tackle a cancer – are without evidence. Some actually have very successful research behind them – and even clinical trials. We will look into 4 of them to see what we can learn:

- The Gerson Therapy
- The Hoxsey Therapy
- The Gonzalez Therapy
- The Pfeifer Protocol

CHAPTER 10
THE APPLIANCE OF SCIENCE

'*The secret of success is consistency of purpose*', said Benjamin Disraeli. Nowhere can this be more true than with Dr Nicholas Gonzalez, a doctor practising in New York, and with Professor Ben Pfeifer in Switzerland, each with clinical trials to support their disciplined and detailed Diet Therapies.

Dr Nicholas Gonzalez

Dr Nicholas Gonzalez has treated cancer patients for nearly 30 years. His methodology is heavily influenced by the theories of Scottish embryologist **Dr John Beard**, later polished and developed by William Kelley.

When studying the foetus in the womb back in 1906, Beard observed that the placenta stopped growing on the precise day the pancreas of the foetus became active and started to secrete its own enzymes (around day 56). He concluded that since there was no logic to the foetus needing pancreatic enzymes to aid digestion (nutrition being provide by the mother via the placenta in a pre-digested form), the enzymes must have another role.

Beard noticed that placental cells (trophoblast cells derived from stem cells) acted rather like cancer cells, and hypothesised that if pancreatic enzymes could stop them growing, maybe they could do the same for cancer. He also noted that around day 56 the first signs of structure started to appear in the foetus – the rapidly growing blob of stem cells was now developing ear, eye and organ cells. Maybe pancreatic enzymes could take rapidly dividing stem cells and turn them into normal, slower growing body cells?

So his theory was simple. A stem cell under the influence of oestrogen, the female hormone, produces a trophoblast cell. This can divide rapidly and is essentially the same as a cancer cell. Pancreatic enzymes can 'convert' this into a normal cell. 102 years ago he even suggested that maybe cancer was like having a baby growing in the wrong place at the wrong time! He wrote a book *'The Enzyme Theory of Cancer'* but after his death in 1923 and, with the emergence of techniques like the radiation work of Marie Curie and then chemotherapy, his work was simply forgotten.

Until in 1970 a dentist, **Dr William Donald Kelley** was looking for something to help him with his wife's breast cancer. He followed Beard's theories and cured his wife with a dietary programme that included pancreatic enzymes. Kelley believed that cancer progressed because of a lack of cancer digesting enzymes in the body and that the pancreas was the prime cancer fighting organ in the body.

After treating his wife successfully he decided to open a clinic and treated 455 patients with some 26 different cancers successfully over a 20 year period. His treatment programme had 5 parts:

- **Nutritional Therapy** – to break down the cancer cells; megavitamins, minerals, high dose vitamin C, bioflavenoids, coenzymes, raw almonds, amino acids and raw beef formula with pancreatic enzymes.
- **Detoxification** – to cleanse the liver and body of dead cells; laxative purges, Epsom Salts, fasts, lemon juice, coffee enemas.
- **Diet** – to rebalance the body and the immune system. (At the outset he felt this needed to be strictly vegetarian but over time changed that view.) He majored on organic foods like nuts (including almonds) and seeds, low protein grains, and raw fruits and vegetables. He avoided processed foods, pesticide residues, refined foods, peanuts and dairy.
- **Neurological Stimulation** – to allow free flow of the body energy to the cancer site, he advocated osteopaths, chiropractors and physiotherapists.
- **Spiritual** – Kelley urged patients to read the Bible, to trust in God and to pray.

Kelley changed his views on a vegetarian diet believing in the end that everybody has their own personal 'metabolic code' and that this code determines what foods best nourish that person. He developed his own 'malignancy system' with 10 different 'Metabolic' or Dietary Types, and 95 variations within those. He recorded his Treatment Programme and case histories in a book, *'One Answer to Cancer'*.

Bill Wolcott, who had also followed the work of Dr John Beard and worked with Kelley has developed this Metabolic Typing further still, using nine controls including blood types, endocrine levels, prostaglandin levels, electrolyte levels and more. He claims to have helped over 60,000 people nourish their bodies maximally using his typing programme. You can even go a long way towards the full service he offers on the web: Try: www.healthexcel.com.

Gonzalez became interested in Kelley's work whilst a student at Cornell University Medical School in 1981. As part of his fourth year thesis he reviewed Kelley's work and then turned it into a formal two year project. In his research, Gonzalez tracked 50 of Kelley's patients, all of whom had been originally given a poor prognosis, but all subsequently enjoyed long-term survival after adopting Kelley's regime.

He also reviewed the case histories of 22 patients with pancreatic cancer – a cancer where 5-year survival in America is just 4 per cent. After interviewing the patients themselves, plus families of the deceased and reviewing medical records, his very thorough final report was met with scorn because, as many experts now believe, Kelley's work had clearly out-performed orthodox treatments. In 1986, Kelley decided to retire – and Gonzalez took up the mantle. Gonzalez now works in New York, not just on cancer but on all manner of diseases. He was joined by Dr Linda Isaacs in 1985.

In 1993 the Associate Director of Cancer Therapy in the NCI invited him to present his work across all cancers. Uniquely the NCI has sponsored a full three phase clinical trial on his work. This was monitored by the FDA and his work paid for ($1.4 million) by the American National Institute of Health's National Centre for Complementary and Alternative Medicine. He has focused on pancreatic cancer in the trials because it is so hard to beat, and results might occur more quickly and noticeably.

In the preliminary studies patients undertaking the Gonzalez regime lived on average 17.5 months – or three times longer than those taking the orthodox medical approach. In further trials,

126 patients were treated with the FDA approved drug gemcitabine. No-one lived past month 19. In the Gonzalez Regime, despite 8 of his 11 patients starting out with grade 4 disease, 5 of the 11 survived 24 months, 2 actually more than 48 months. Gonzalez doesn't just want to cure people though. He wants his 'Dietary' regime thoroughly tested and incorporated as standard practice within orthodox mainstream medicine. Political Dynamite!

The Gonzalez regime has three basic parts:

1. **Detoxification** – involving a variety of cleanses and two coffee enemas each day.
2. **Diet** – individually designed diets as a result of extensive metabolic typing. Diets avoid refined, processed and prepared foods. Some patients are encouraged to become vegans, others to eat meat, depending upon personal metabolism traits.
3. **Supplementation** – 120 to 175 supplements may be used daily, again, tailored to the individual's requirements. These involve trace minerals, antioxidants and pancreatic enzymes.

If nothing else, Gonzalez' work exposes the UK orthodox medical 'quacks' who say that there is no evidence that changing your diet can possibly beat cancer. You can find far more detail on our web site, and in my book, *'Conventional Cancer Cures – What's the Alternative?'*

Professor Ben Pfeifer

Another person with clinical trials behind their Diet Therapy is Professor Ben Pfeifer at the Aeskulap Clinic in Switzerland. Although Pfeifer started with prostate cancer patients, he is now moving on to other hormonally driven cancers.

Pfeifer's Protocol was primarily developed for hormone refractory prostate cancer – a state where the patient had little hope of long-term cure. Clinical studies show Pfeifer's treatment programme has a 65 per cent success rate, even though it has been used largely with patients for whom orthodox treatment has failed. His work was covered originally in the Swiss Journal of Oncology, January 2005.

Pfeifer uses an individually tailored programme of herbs, glyconutrients, minerals and vitamins. All these are centred on four commercially developed products:

- **Prostasol** – containing herbs such as saw palmetto, pygeum, reishi, ginger, nettles, skullcap, beta-sitosterol, and is licensed in Holland with no tainting from oestrogenic products.
- **Biobran** – is a natural food extract, made from 'pre-digested' rice bran using enzymes from shitake mushrooms. It is a powerful immune system booster which works by stimulating the activity of T- and B-lymphocytes and Natural Killer cells – the front line in your body's defences. There are over 15 published studies in science journals on this immuno-modulator, highlighting its safety and effectiveness in individuals who have compromised immune systems.
- **Imupros** – is a blend of nutritional supplements including vitamins, trace elements, ginseng, lycopene and green tea extract.
- **Curcumin Complex** – is a mix of **curcumin**, a potent anti-inflammatory and antioxidant compound found in the spice turmeric; and **resveratrol**, a strong antioxidant, plant compound from red grapes; and **black pepper** which enhances absorption.

Interestingly, Pfeifer's protocol doesn't deliver where the patient's cancer is not oestrogen driven, nor when radiotherapy has caused damage.

Although the standard UK orthodox medical line is to ignore the Swiss clinical trials, one hospital – St Bartholomew's Hospital, London – is at least honest enough to say that, in the absence of any worthwhile treatments for this late stage prostate cancer, they may as well give the Pfeifer Protocol a try. It's not an official trial – and certainly not a clinical trial – and only about a dozen patients have been allowed to take up the full Protocol, to see if it provides any benefit. You can read far more on our web site, where we will include updates.

Pfeifer, meanwhile, is now developing his Protocol for other cancer types.

What is common between Gonzalez and Pfeifer, apart from the fact that their programmes are supported in clinical research, is that the exact programme is tailored to you and your cancer, and both involve very detailed testing, and then a very large number of highly active ingredients given with specific purpose to meet specific needs.

The Gerson Therapy

Guaranteed to make certain orthodox medical experts turn puce purely at its mention, the Gerson Therapy has no such clinical trials behind it. Just a number of people who are alive today, when modern medicine predicted otherwise.

The Gerson Therapy was developed by Dr Max Gerson (1881–1959) for migraine but he noted it had an effect with TB, and so started to treat people in the 1920s for an incurable form of TB, where he achieved phenomenal results. The Gerson Therapy is more than just a diet therapy – it is a healing discipline. Although primarily used by people who already have a chronic illness, it is however occasionally used in a preventative context. It may well be hard work but, for some, the effort is truly worthwhile.

> *"Suffering isn't ennobling, recovery is."*
> (Dr Christiaan Barnard).

Let us be quite clear. For a number of people, and many of those for whom orthodox medicine had failed, the Gerson Therapy has been an important part of their 'recovery'. There are many anecdotes, most notably Oxford Don Michael Gearin-Tosh, and Beata Bishop, two of the people who more than beat the odds with the Gerson Therapy. Michael lived 10 full years after being diagnosed with terminal multiple myeloma – sadly he died recently of something completely unrelated. Beata turned to the therapy 22 years ago with her melanoma when all the orthodox treatments had failed her. You can find much more on our web site.

The basic principle behind the therapy is to heal the whole body by returning the body systems, key organs and cells to the state they should be in, if you had a healthy non-toxic body. The net aim is twofold: The stimulation of the body's own immune defences to do what they normally do in a healthy body, plus the readjustment in the balance of the molecules and atoms within the cells, returning them to levels normally found in healthy cells. It is a healing, restorative strategy for all diseases, not merely cancer.

Once both parts of this therapy are fully established the theory is that a diseased body will simply restore itself to full health – just as nature intended. There is no doubt that this therapy has had notable successes, especially given that patients tend to be in later stages of their cancer, having often tried and failed with all available orthodox treatments beforehand.

However, diseased cancer cells frequently liquefy, which in itself creates a further problem. The process of breaking down tumours can be so effective that large amounts of toxins are released into the bloodstream by the diseased cells. (It should be noted that patients frequently experience 'healing reactions' when these large amounts of toxins are released from the cells into the blood system.)

However, as I covered earlier, the largest detoxification organ, namely the liver, is often seriously toxic itself and simply cannot treat the sudden increases in toxins flooding into the blood stream. So it needs help – it needs to be cleansed itself, and super-charged to help it better eliminate all the extra toxins.

One method of achieving this is to stimulate the liver with up to five coffee enemas per day for a limited period, whilst using castor oil every other day. This causes increases in the levels of bile juices, and a dilation of the bile ducts, themselves, making the passage of toxins easier.

Dr Max Gerson was described by Dr Albert Schweitzer as, *one of the most eminent geniuses in medical history."* He originally published *A Cancer Therapy: Results of Fifty Cases,* over fifty years ago. His work is now driven by his eighty-something year old daughter Charlotte, who stresses that it the therapy is applicable to a host of diseases, not merely cancer, and that even healthy people should consider a period on the therapy from time to time merely as a precautionary detox.

Officially, the therapy aims to provide optimum nutrition consisting of a deliberate over abundance of minerals, enzymes and vitamins, whilst avoiding the toxic pesticides and herbicides of normal food by using only organic versions.

The basic principles of the therapy are:

- The use of only organic food to avoid pesticide and herbicide toxins.
- Very limited fat and protein consumption both of which are known to 'feed' cancer cells – no animal fat or protein in the first eight weeks; nor milk and soya.
- No pulses (lentils, beans and, again, soya) to be consumed as they can prevent mineral uptake because of their phytic acid content. (NB. You could just skim this off the surface of the boiled pulses though.)
- All water used for cooking or rinsing must be provided from distilled or reverse osmosis sources.
- Water must not be drunk as it dilutes the power of the juices. A little peppermint tea is allowed.
- Neither plastic nor tin foil may be used as it may contaminate food.
- The diet is limited to – 1) freshly made juices of vegetables, fruits and leaves, consumed within 20 minutes of preparation to avoid losses in enzyme effectiveness and 2) large quantities of raw fruit and vegetables, along with some lightly steamed vegetables, stewed fruit, potatoes and oatmeal.
- Organic, in season, fresh vegetables and fruit are the ideal.

The aim is to exclude sodium, whilst dramatically increasing potassium intake as we discussed in Chapter 3. Fresh juices provide more easily absorbed and digested nutrients, whilst not taxing the impaired body systems. The use of hourly juices over the length of the day also avoids calorie and, thus, insulin surges and actually limits the total number of calories consumed per day.

Absolutely **essential** to the diet therapy are:

- Apples – raw.
- Carrots – raw and lightly cooked.
- Potatoes – baked, mashed or in potato salad.
- Sweet potatoes – but only once per week.
- Fresh fruit – grapes, cherries, mangoes, peaches, oranges, apricots, grapefruit, banana, tangerines, pears, plums, melons, papayas (pears and plums may be stewed).
- Dried fruit – apricots, dates, figs, peaches, raisins, prunes.

Absolutely **forbidden** are:

- All things bottled, canned, frozen, preserved, refined, salted, smoked and sulphured.
- Bicarbonate of soda in food, toothpaste and mouthwashes.
- Alcohol.
- Salts.
- Avocado (too much fatty acid).
- Basil, oregano (aromatic oils can cause difficult reactions).
- Berries (except red, black and whole currants).
- Biscuits, cake, chocolate, cocoa, coffee (any sort), tea.
- Cucumbers.
- Fats and oils (except flaxseed),
- Mushrooms, nuts (too much fatty acids/fats), peas (sulphured), lentils, beans, seeds (phytic acid/enzyme inhibitors).
- Pickles.
- Pineapples.
- Refined flour.
- Soft drinks, fizzy and fruit juices (preserved).
- Soya (fat content and phytic acid).
- Spices.
- Sugar (including sweets).
- Tap water.

Forbidden for first eight weeks: all dairy, eggs, meat and fish.

The type of juicer is also crucial. Centrifugal juicers simply do not get the full volumes of minerals, vitamins and enzymes out. Gerson recommended a heavy press juicer that involves two stages and a double press.

The therapy is arduous. A ten-hour day spent juicing plus making and using the coffee enemas is not unusual; and a period of two years to fully cleanse the body is not uncommon. The theory is that it takes a long time for the body to develop the many stages of the cancer process in the first place, and so it takes an equally long time to get rid of them all to restore everything to maximum working order!

So the therapy is hard work. You need time to prepare the fresh juices, as they have to be drunk at their prime. Then there is the preparation and use of the coffee enemas. But as Goethe said, *"The day is of infinite length for him who knows how to appreciate and use it."*

The Gerson Institute has been criticised in the past for not adapting the therapy as new scientific discoveries were made for natural compounds. This has now been addressed and there is even a new book out from Charlotte Gerson and that covers the issue: *Healing – The Gerson Way.*

Other elements of the therapy:

Gerson used crude **liver extract** to boost his patients liver function, but nowadays this extract is more refined and seems not so potent. While Gerson used his own calves liver preparation, most sources now seem to have pesticide residues and campylobacter infection. **Coenzyme Q 10** and defatted **colostrum** (the first fluid secreted in a mother's breast) are now used to boost the immune system.

Pancreatic enzymes have always been a part of the therapy, as have **WobeMugos tablets** containing a number of anti-tumour and immune boosting natural compounds.

Recent additions have included the use of **hyperthermia, B-17** and **ozone therapy.** Supplements like **grapefruit seed extract, Pau D'Arco, selenium** and **chromium picolinate** (which stimulates the pancreas) are also now used. Some critics claim that the loss of the liver extract is major – I have no evidence one way or the other.

What I do observe is that the current therapy is not as random as some critics suggest. Blood tests monitoring all manner of enzyme, toxin and mineral levels are taken on a frequent basis, and adjustments are made as a result.

The Plaskett Therapy

One of the Gerson-needs-to-be-updated critics was Dr Lawrence Plaskett, formerly vice chair of the UK Nutritional Cancer Therapy Trust. After a degree in biochemistry at Cambridge, a doctorate at London University and a number of years in food companies and government agencies, Dr Plaskett turned his extensive knowledge to updating the Gerson Therapy. He now educates new nutritionists to degree level.

His research on natural compounds in food is extremely detailed. Plaskett in the UK and John Boik in the USA really do expose the lack of knowledge inherent in British Orthodox Medicine on this subject.

Plaskett argues that many recent scientific discoveries have proven that Gerson was totally right and considerably 'ahead of his time'. The latest scientific studies have supported, for example, the importance of omega 3 (from fish oils and linseed oil) as an essential element in the good health of cells; the use of coffee enemas to induce raised levels of glutathione S-transferases, the enzymes of liver detoxification; the use of high potassium in the diet and digestive enzymes to help increase absorption.

Where he feels recent studies have added to Gerson is that there is no need for castor oil, iodine and iodide, dried thyroid, liver juices and liver injections. Instead he recommends a very detailed and precise list of supplements, some of which vary according to the cancer.

Plaskett's version of t/he therapy is vigorously vegan. Dairy products, eggs, fish and meat are excluded, because he argues that cancers thrive on protein and a low protein diet has been shown to be effective against cancer (Tannenbaum).

Plaskett is also a firm believer in the eat-to-beat-cancer principle and it is his firmly held view that a nutritional approach to cancer should be nationally available. There are at least 90 trained Plaskett Therapists throughout the UK.

Notable Others

I could tell you about **Dr Contreras at the Oasis of Hope** in Mexico (Contreras is Mexican). He uses a modified version of the Gerson Therapy; plus 'Metabolic Therapy' consisting of B-17 treatment along with pancreatic enzymes, vitamin C megadoses, spiritual healing and prayer. He can use chemotherapy and radio-therapy too (*'I just don't find it works as well'*, he says). Or **Dr David Walker,** a university physics professor who developed colon cancer and cured himself by a disciplined combination of diet, supplements, oxygenating programmes and his own cellular re-energising system, based on his knowledge of physics, to get the cells working properly again. He formed a clinic, helped thousands of patients and was hounded out of America to his current home in Mexico.

There are many others – check out our web site.

Summary

> *"Despair is the price one pays for setting oneself an impossible aim."*
> (Graham Greene)

If you have cancer, curing yourself through a diet therapy is certainly not an impossible aim.

There are a number of similarities between the above thera-pies.

Firstly, patients tend to only use these therapies at a late stage of the cancer – often when orthodox medical approaches have failed. Despite this, the clinical trials and the anecdotes tell a posi-tive story.

Secondly, they are often disciplined, involving detailed blood and biochemical analysis.

Thirdly, the Diet Therapies are not vegetarian – they may use metabolic typing to determine whether meat should be consumed or not; or they may be 'fat and protein' free – thus eliminating everything from dairy to soya to meat and fish. It's a moot point but an important one.

Finally, they all have width. They don't rely on a couple of vitamins, or a vegetarian diet or giving up alcohol. They have a total concept – something to tackle the whole cancer process. For example:

- Boosting the immune system with natural compounds.
- Correcting mineral imbalances and deficiencies.
- Trying to return the cells to a healthy normal state.
- Using natural compounds to attack the cancer cells.
- Using natural compounds (like fish oils) to reduce inflammation.
- Using pancreatic enzymes to try to turn off the cancer cells.

As you can see it is totally wrong to suggest changing your diet doesn't make a jot of difference – it can save your life.

The issue is, if you don't want to take yourself off to New York, California, Switzerland or Mexico, how can you construct a layman's version of these than can tackle the diversity of the whole cancer process?

CHAPTER 11
ACID AND ALKALINE BODIES

I receive a lot of letters and e mails. Quite a few ask about foods to restore an alkaline body. I need to correct some mythology here and now.

A neutral non-acid, non-alkaline solution has a pH of 7.0, on a scale of zero (acid) to 14 (alkaline). The human body works best when its pH is between 7.2 and 7.4, which means it is very slightly alkaline.

A number of health books will tell you two things which are true, and two things that are rubbish.

1. There are a number of foods and lifestyle factors which are acid making:
    For example:
    > Sugar
    > Chocolate
    > Salt
    > Vinegar
    > Tobacco
    > Stress
    > Refined flour
    > Processed foods
    > Prepared foods
    > Chinese food.
2. There are a number of foods and lifestyle factors that are alkali producing:
    > Most fresh fruits – apples, pears, grapes etc
    > Most fresh vegetables – greens, broccoli, garlic, radishes
    > Most herbs.
3. The factors that cause acidity are far greater than the factors that cause alkalinity.
4. This is due to acid ash or alkaline ash residue being produced in the stomach.

I have even been taken in myself by some of this – and I apologise to my readers if I have misled them in the past and seem to be going back on myself.

The first myth is this 'acid/alkaline ash in the stomach' rubbish. It is simply not true. I've seen books that include bananas, plums, prunes and oranges in the acid ash making category – and that is nonsense too. Or lemons in the alkali group and oranges and grapefruit in the acid group. Nonsense. I've written to two of the biggest exponents of the theory and they have come back with no evidence at all.

Anyway, the acid and alkali levels in the body and importantly in your cells simply do not 'work' like this.

Acid and alkali bodies – the truth

- **Potassium and magnesium rich foods will help make your cells alkaline** – as we have told you – and in turn your immune system and all your organs will become alkaline. And your body will thrive.

  The biggest sources of potassium and magnesium have already been covered but principally they include all fruits and all vegetables (bananas, oranges, plums are excellent potassium sources – as are tomatoes, asparagus, Brussel sprouts and rhubarb which are often included in this acid ash list), herbs, whole grains, whole rice and fresh nuts and seeds.

- **Anything that directly reduces the cells potassium levels and increases the sodium levels will make your cells more acid.** And this is a bad thing.

  > MSG and Chinese foods
  > Salt
  > Sugar
  > Processed foods
  > Prepared foods
  > Smoked foods
  > Dried meats, salamis, pates, sausages, bacon

- **Other foods and lifestyle factors can have indirect effects** – for example on hormones – and this will have a knock on effect making your cells more acid.

  > Tobacco
  > Dairy
  > Stress
  > Preservatives, pesticides, toiletries, household cleaners – anything that contains toxins and especially chemicals that mimic the action of oestrogen (like toluene in nail polishes and perfumes)
  > Poor sleeping patterns
  > Hormone supplements that increase levels of oestrogen
  > A lack of beneficial bacteria in the intestine

- By and large, **the factors that make your cells acid are more powerful than those that make them more alkaline.** The acid debits – of stress, sugar, salt etc – tend to have stronger effects than the alkali credits – eating a pear or an apple. So if you are 'acid' you have to work harder to restore yourself to full health.

I hope this clears up some of the mythology coming from certain 'Alternative' health practitioners.

CHAPTER 12

CLEAN WATER –
THE ONLY SOLUTION

As JB Haldane once exclaimed, *'Even the Archbishop of Canterbury is 85 per cent water!'*

If a plant in your garden is drooping and limp, you may add nutrients to the soil and you will certainly add water. But, if the water is contaminated you know the plant will be affected. Why do you not use this thinking with your own health?

Clean water is essential to our health. It affects all our cells, our enzymatic processes and our ability to detox, and treatments such as the Gerson Therapy stress the use of pure water for cancer patients, even for cooking and washing utensils.

Remember – you drink tap water and you bathe in it. And the skin is not a barrier, as some water companies would ask us to believe. It is a carrier. If it were not, how would a nicotine or oestrogen patch work?

We suspect our tap water is less than perfect but are told that individual pollutants are below Government determined safe levels, so we have no need to worry. And the whole issue on water safety ends up in a dispute between logic and statistics. Governments may feel there is little evidence that individual pollutants may be causing problems, but it seems logical that the combined effects may be far worse.

Rain falling brings with it smoke, dust, chemical fumes, germs, lead and strontium 90 to name but a few things. The Swedes blame the UK industrial revolution for clouds of acid rain that wiped out the fish population in some of their lakes.

Water then flows through the soil, in rivers and streams picking up fertilisers, pesticides, herbicides and nitrates.

Some people buy organic food only then to cook it in tap water; or they make their decaffeinated herb tea with boiled tap water. Boiling merely concentrates certain contaminants.

Back to basics – the need for water?

The late Dr Batmanghelidj, formally of St Mary's Hospital Medical School (part of Imperial College, London), provided a strong case for drinking at least two litres of water a day in his book, *'Your Body's Many Cries for Water'*. He argued very convincingly that dehydration can be responsible for a huge range of ailments and degenerative diseases including dyspeptic pain, rheumatoid arthritis pain, stress and depression, high blood pressure, high blood cholesterol, excess body weight, asthma and allergies. He showed how these diseases and ailments often originate from metabolic stress, and one of the biggest contributory factors to this stress is dehydration.

In the author's postscript, he added, *'When will all NHS doctors start looking at dehydration and getting their patients to increase their clean water consumption?'*

Others will argue that two litres of water per day per adult is an absolute minimum for proper cellular hydration, with three litres probably closer to the mark if we exercise or we are ill, having radiotherapy treatment and so on.

But what is the science? When I was in advertising I once asked a famous bottled water company for their support to the need for two litres per day – and they told me that they had none.

The FSA in the UK achieve a figure of 8 glasses a day based on an analysis of how much water you use in an average day, less the water you consume when eating foods such as fruit and vegetables. On average, the body loses 1-1.5 litres of water per day, more if you exercise, more if you are in a hot climate.

Too much water can actually reduce levels of salts and important electrolytes in the body. In **icon** we covered the story of a London Theatre artist who sang and danced his way through a two-hour performance every night. He regularly drank 14 bottles of water a night and ended up in hospital with total electrolyte imbalance!

In April 2008 doctors in the Renal Division of the University of Pennsylvania have concluded in the Journal of American Society of Nephrology that there is no evidence whatsoever for the claims that 2 litres or more will help you detoxify or help you lose weight or avoid headaches and so on. They do say that drinking more water will help clear the body of salt and urea but conclude that the issue is to drink 'enough', stating that there is no research showing benefit in drinking larger amounts.

So what is enough? And again the answer is as individual as you are. You may be healthy and normal in a cool climate. You may live up a mountain, or in the tropics, you may be ill and having treatments. The simple way to tell if you are drinking enough water is to check the colour of your urine. It should be almost colourless – a very pale yellow. If you are taking B vitamins, or a multivitamin containing B vitamins, or turmeric/curcumin supplements it will be a little darker.

The rule of thumb is that if you have dark yellow or even brown urine you are simply not drinking enough water. The SAS and top sportsmen use this simple system because they know that a 5 per cent drop in body liquids causes tiredness and sluggishness, which can reduce performance by 50 per cent.

The toxins in water

If you have cancer, it is crucial to try to establish what caused the cancer so you can make every attempt to cut it out of your life. What if that toxin were water-borne?

Prime areas of concern in tap water supplies are:

- Chlorine and fluorine
- Heavy metals
- Pesticides, fertilisers and herbicides
- Drugs and oestrogens.

In an Iowa study (Lynch, Zhang, Olsen) there were significantly higher levels of female lung cancer and male bladder cancer in towns with surface water supply and shadow wells. Pesticides and other chemicals on the land were implicated.

Chlorine is added to water, for example, to kill germs and bacteria, but it also destroys vitamin E and kills the 'friendly bacteria' in the intestinal tract. Chlorine can damage arteries and can even oxidise other contaminants in the water to produce free radicals or, worse, combine to produce chloroform, chloramines and other toxic by-products, which are carcinogenic.

The National Research Council in the USA has prepared a 379 page report on trichloroethylene. Always known to be a dangerous pollutant and linked to child leukaemia, kidney cancer and a number of illnesses, the report concludes that TCE is actually 40 times more powerful than originally thought! And levels of TCE have been increasing in tap water as chlorine combines with other increasing levels of pollutants. These two new discoveries mean that in certain regions the water TCE content is now actually above the original safety levels set by the Government.

Another research study published in May 2008 by researchers at Birmingham University analysed birth defects in babies born between 2001 and 2003 in Taiwan, where chlorine levels are almost identical to those in tap water in the UK. They found a doubling in birth defects like hole-in-the-heart, cleft palates, urinary tract defects, brain defects and Down's syndrome. Earlier studies have linked chlorinated water to miscarriage, still birth and bladder cancer. The researchers identified trihalomethanes (THM's) as the cause – and stated that you can increase levels in the womb by drinking the water, or bathing in it.

In a Finnish study on surface water (*AMJ* August 1999), chlorinated water was linked to increased incidences of bladder, kidney and stomach cancers. The US Environmental Agency has stated that prolonged and frequent swimming in chlorinated pools contributes to skin cancer (*Epidemiology* 1992: 3). Chlorinated water also contributes to miscarriages (*JAWWA* 1992: 20) and gastrointestinal cancer, bladder cancer and rectal cancer (*American Journal of Public Health* 1997: 87).

Some 1000 cities now treat their water with ozone, which has had a significant effect on purity.

Fluoride: Fluoride is an acknowledged 'equivocal carcinogen'. It was downgraded (for reasons beyond my comprehension) a few years back from 'clear evidence of carcinogenicity'.

All the original tests used by Governments worldwide to encourage fluoridation of water purported to show that fluorine was a tooth and bone protecting agent. Calcium fluoride was the proposed additive. Approval was given on that basis.

But life moves on and now in the UK we use sodium fluoride, formerly used as a rat poison and a by-product of the aluminium industry, which causes it to be contaminated by metals such as aluminium and even arsenic. This water treatment is illegal in Sweden, Denmark and Holland, since apparently sodium fluoride contains too many heavy metals, and anyway fluoride can inhibit thyroid function and damage the immune system. Hypothyroidism is a definite consequence of too much fluoride.

While Governments and water companies add chlorine to water to treat water, they add fluoride to water to treat people. Without our consent.

It is medically contra-indicated – for pregnant mothers (US Government, 1966), formula-fed infants, diabetics and people with kidney impairment.

It's not as if we don't get enough fluoride in this modern world. Sulphuryl fluoride, for example, is used as a fumigant on nuts, wheat and over 150 US foodstuffs many of which are sold in Britain. Residues on these foods can be 130 times higher than the level in our water. It's a psychotropic drug and the cousin of Prozac.

Worse, toothpastes commonly contain sodium fluoride. In the USA there are on-pack warnings which read, '*As with all fluoride toothpastes, keep out of the reach of children under 6 years of age. If you do accidentally swallow more than used for brushing, seek professional assistance or contact a poison control officer immediately*'.

There is virtually no hard evidence that fluoridation improves children's teeth, indeed, quite the opposite. Teotia and Teotia conducted the largest dental study in the world in India. Over 30 years, they examined 400,000 children and found that tooth decay increased with fluoride concentrations in the water and decreased with calcium concentration.

In the USA, The National Institute of Environmental Health Sciences is currently investigating a Harvard professor who was sponsored to the tune of $13 million to look into child bone cancer and fluoridation. He actually reported to Federal Officials on his study that no link between child bone cancer and fluoridation was found. However, when the full report arrived, the detail showed there was clearly a risk, especially to boys of a young age! His links to the toothpaste companies are also being investigated.

Aluminium: is present in significant quantities in tap water, as it can be added to clarify the water during treatment. A detailed review paper published in March 2002 discussed the powerful evidence showing that aluminium from drinking water and other sources is a major contributory factor to Alzheimer's disease, which is becoming increasingly common amongst older people.

Adding insult to injury, research shows that aluminium can react with low-doses of fluoride in water, causing more aluminium to cross the blood-brain barrier and become deposited in the brain. Julie Varner and her colleagues showed this definitively in a detailed 52-week study of rats, published in the prestigious peer-reviewed journal *Brain Research*. Aluminium is a potent neurotoxin and has also been implicated as a co-factor in the initiation of cancer.

Other metals: Old pipes in the water system and chemicals deposited in streams can lead to **lead, mercury** and **copper** contamination. Mercury's negatives are well chronicled; both lead and copper inhibit zinc uptake in the body and zinc is important in a variety of ways from enhancing vitamin C effectiveness to protecting against prostate cancers. One theory of prostate cancer is that low levels of zinc are linked to heavy metal displacement.

The National Academy of Sciences (September 2001) showed that even very low levels of **arsenic** in the water were linked to cancer (the United States EPA set standards in 1975 and may well have them wrong was the conclusion). Studies have been made from China to Chile and arsenic is increasingly found to seep into the soil from natural sources, agriculture and industrial waste.

Parasites are now common in 20 per cent of the British population. In Carolina 82 per cent of the population were getting theirs from the water system as the microscopic parasites had become immune to chlorine.

Nitrate and nitrite: A study of 22,000 women in Iowa showed that **nitrate**, common in rural areas was associated with bladder cancer. 20 per cent of ingested nitrate was shown to be transformed in the body to nitrite and N-nitroso compounds causing cancers such as colon and bladder (May 2001 study).

Scientists from 19 countries at IARC in Lyon (2007) have concluded that high **nitrite** levels, especially in conjunction with low vitamin C levels are linked to various cancers especially stomach, oesophagael and brain. Of special concern was the run off of water from pesticides in the fields, with nitrates and nitrites either directly promoting cancer through the water supplies or indirectly via the by-products of their effect on cyanobacteria in the soil.

Radon: The National Association of Scientists in America in 1998 showed that radon in the water supply was linked to lung cancers. Radon can leach into water supplies where the underlying rock contains even small uranium deposits. This is a potential risk in some areas of South West and North West England.

Drugs: Another debate concerns **oestrogen** levels in the recycled drinking water of major cities, originating from ladies who take HRT and contraceptive pills. This has been blamed for reduced fertility, and for increases in testicular cancer. Sperm count is down 20 per cent in the UK in 25 years, whilst testicular cancer is up 80 per cent. It has also been blamed for male fish showing female organ development and young human male offspring developing testicle problems and even reducing penis size. Hormones are very powerful substances – they can work in concentrations of less than one part per billion, the sort of levels it is almost impossible to selectively remove from water.

(The counter claim is that in Denmark and Scotland, where there is no use of recycled water, oestrogen levels in the populations are also rising. The blame is put on a variety of chemicals in the environment, particularly endocrine (hormone) disrupters like chemical oestrogen mimics (xenoestrogens), for example from white lined cans, plastic bottles, even plastic children's toys, and plastic wrapped food and plastics in general. Certain plasticisers are worse than others and one really has no idea whether the plastic bottle or cup in front of you is harmless or dangerous. Recent US research showed that where a hot liquid was used in a plastic container made of certain plasticisers, harmful chemicals were released at a 40-fold increased level, and continued to be so even on subsequent use of cold liquids. Then there are xenoestrogens from petrol fumes, cleaning agents, toiletries and detergents, as we covered previously.)

Whatever the reason, the issue is: 'Do these harmful chemicals get into your drinking water?' Roger Lilley of Friends of the Earth blames a lack of monitoring by water companies, particularly on local rivers. Both the river Aire in Scotland and the river Lee (from where London gets drinking water) are, in varying degrees, already toxic to wildlife, according to Friends of the Earth.

Nowadays with our increased use of **drugs** (like steroids and antibiotics; or Tamoxifen and statins both of which have recently been shown to remain active in the body for more than 5 years) combined with the increasing numbers of old people who already consume over 60 per cent of all drugs in the UK, synthetic oestrogen is not the only drug that potentially could make it into a big city's water supply. Is it enough to hope that all these drugs are removed in your recycled drinking water?

Action?

What are we to do? What is increasingly clear is that there is no such thing as 'generic' tap water, only 'local' tap water. The concentrations of different potential carcinogens vary greatly by region and many are not totally removed under normal conditions. The issue isn't just about drinking of course. You wash your vegetables in it, and your cups and plates. You cook in it. You bathe the baby in it.

Plastic bottled water is increasingly felt to be less than perfect because of the plasticisers I talked about above, potentially leaching from the plastic into the water. These can be carcinogenic even in minute quantities and as Dr Anna Soto of Tufts showed, they can be cumulative.

Boiling the water merely increases the concentration of the toxins dissolved.

Distillation, if you had the time and the apparatus, can work, but it is hard to provide enough volume for all your rinsing and cooking needs on top of water levels for drinking.

The most convenient way of removing contaminants is through **filtration**. A double carbon filter can be installed under the sink. It is relatively cheap, but seems to be rather limited in its filtration abilities.

Then there is a **reverse osmosis water filter.**

The great advantage of this system is that you eliminate nearly all of the fluoride, parasites and bacteria, oestrogen, chlorine and aluminium in your drinking water, as well as a host of other potentially toxic chemicals, hormone disrupters and drugs, as long as you change the filters regularly. If you just measure the more common impurities (in parts per million), a recent test I witnessed showed scores of:

Tap water	400–700
Jug filtered tap water	275
Plastic bottled mineral water	175
Reverse osmosis filtered	6

And therein lies the problem. With reverse osmosis you remove virtually everything – including the minerals that are important for your good health. These minerals are normally dissolved in water and as a result it has a pH of about 7.2. So you see natural water is slightly alkaline, reflected in the ideal body pH which is also slightly alkaline. However, remove all the minerals and you don't just remove potential 'nourishment', you make the water much more acidic. One man in Ireland I know measured his water's pH after reverse osmosis at 5.2.

There has been a lot of press comment and concern about this 'dead' water issue. You could 'compensate' a little by doubling your daily intake of minerals. But you might still miss certain trace elements.

The counter argument is that reverse osmosis water has been consumed throughout South East Asia for the last 25 years without any apparent ill effects. There are mass market machines outside apartment blocks – you simply put a coin in a slot and you fill up your very large plastic container! The big beer companies like Singha, and also Nestlé and Coca Cola have all launched brands of this 'Clean, drinking water.' In both plastic and glass bottles.

Another, more recent idea is a **water ioniser,** with claims that it filters the water effectively, keeps it alkaline and keeps it 'alive'. Unfortunately these currently cost around £700 although doubtless the prices will come down as they become more popular.

For now the most cost effective solution is probably glass bottled water to drink, if you can get it (restaurants can), and use a reverse osmosis filter to provide the inert water for washing and cooking the vegetables and washing the dishes.

Whether you already have cancer or are keen to prevent it, you should take a realistic view of the above facts and plan your action. Water is vital to your body and good health; you simply don't need the impurities it comes with.

CHAPTER 13
CUTTING OUT THE BAD GUYS

Yes, I'm sorry. I did say that other diet books told you what to avoid and cut out and implied this book was going to be different.

My personal view is that you don't have to deprive yourself of all your favourite foods – and I do believe a little of what you fancy does you good. But nonetheless, if there is top quality evidence against certain foods, it is my duty to tell you and your right to know.

Dairy

The White Lies report handed to the UK Government by a team of experts in 2007, in the words of the UK press, 'hammered' dairy. I have been warning readers for 6 years now.

In 2002, the Karolinska Institute produced an epidemiology study, (the same type as the one from which people concluded that smoking cigarettes was linked to increased cancer risk). On the links between dairy consumption and prostate cancer risk, they found a straight line correlation; the more dairy you consume, the greater your risk.

Other studies have shown a less exact, but similar correlation between increased dairy consumption and increased breast cancer risk.

In fact the evidence is almost unarguable against dairy – there have been quite a lot of studies on several different cancers – we have covered them all in **icon**.

For example: 61,000 women were tracked for 13 years in a US study (American Journal of Clinical Nutrition) – a glass of milk a day (or equivalent) doubles ovarian cancer risk.

For example: 5,000 people were followed for 65 years – those children who grew up in families consuming the highest amounts of dairy (two cups per day each) had three times the colorectal cancer risk later in life (Jolieke, Queensland)

And bad news for the British – adding milk to tea ruins the health benefits of tea according to the Charité University

Hospital, Berlin. The cassein (milk protein) content of the milk, sticks to the beneficial polyphenols of the tea and negates them.

People come to me after speeches and ask if consuming low-fat or skimmed milk or organic milk would be alright?

It is true of course that average dairy cow in the USA now produces 50 (yes, 50) times the volume of milk over its predecessors 20 years ago. How? Through hormones, drugs, genetic changes and 'super' feeds, which are often based on animal protein even though cows are herbivores. And the fat in milk is a solvent likely to bring with it all manner of hormones (natural and injected), antibiotics, pesticides and herbicides from the fields, So organic might have less of these toxins in it and low fat might also be much better for you.

But the real problem does not go away with low fat or organic milk. The issue is bigger than drugs or pesticides. It is a hormone, Insulin-like Growth Factor 1 or IGF-1, which helps a baby calf grow to full size in about 10 months. IGF-1 causes cells to grow rapidly, and we humans don't need this turbo-charged growth, in fact it is dangerous. IGF-1 has been shown to cause cancer cell proliferation.

Mosanto, the giant American food company, and the FDA in the USA claim IGF-1 does not cross in any volume from the gut into the bloodstream. Specific Japanese research with mice clearly indicates otherwise.

If that's not enough, as I told you earlier, the high levels of fat and protein in milk prevent absorption of elements like zinc, crucial to vitamin C absorption and action, and also important in the prevention of prostate cancer. Dairy protein and high blood levels of calcium actually reduce magnesium, potassium and vitamin D levels, and prevent the absorption of calcium into tissues and bones. There is increasing evidence that too much blood calcium may even cause cancer, and that vitamin D can help with the prevention and treatment of a number of cancers including colon and breast cancers.

Dairy and its constituents, like cassein and lactose, are found everywhere from biscuits to soups, and it is even contained in some drugs!

Patients fighting cancer do not need high levels of protein and fat in their diets, and nor do they need IGF-1. You should try to cut down on cows' dairy as much as possible. You can get more than enough calcium from a daily helping of 'greens'. A little goat's cheese would be a good replacement for cows' cheese as we have been eating this for longer than and it is more easily digested. You can try rice milk or soya on your cereals. But do not switch your large volume of milk consumption directly for a large volume of soya. Soya has a high fat and protein content too, and for this reason was cut from the Gerson Therapy. Personally I am increasingly concerned about the possible dangers linked to GM soya.

Bad fat

In the Western world, we have two problems with **fats and oils:** We consume too much of them, and we largely consume the wrong sort!

Firstly, fats and oils are basically the same thing. Fat is the solid state, oil is the liquid state.

Next, understand that fat is, anyway, very high in **calories:**

1 gram protein	=	4 calories
1 gram of carbohydrate	=	4 calories
1 gram fat	=	9 calories.

In the USA people regularly consume 50 per cent of their calories as fat, whereas in rural China this figure can be below 10 per cent. And we noted earlier that several research studies show that high calorie consumption can produce more free radicals and lead to more cancer, whereas calorie restriction is an important anti-cancer weapon.

Virtually all fats and oils, when ingested, drive up oestrogen levels. Fats produce steroids, the precursors of oestrogen and oestrogen 'drives' many cancers.

If you don't 'exercise' or burn the excess calories they will be stored as fat, increasing your girth, holding excess hormones and toxins, and limiting your desire and ability to 'move', so setting in a downward spiral.

Next, you probably find it very hard to understand all the

scientific terms surrounding good fats and bad fats – so let me try and explain it simply. In Europe, unless you are living on the Northern shores of the Mediterranean, the majority of fats we consume (and especially the ones our children consume) are **bad** for us.

Saturated and hydrogenated (trans) fats

For many people the great majority of fats and oils they consume are '**hydrogenated**'. This is found in junk food, fast food, chicken nuggets, battered cod, onion rings, bagged snacks, crisps, salted roasted peanuts, processed foods, supermarket bread, biscuits, soup, chips, rice mixes, pasta mixes, pizzas and even some breakfast cereals, health bars and healthy bran-rich products; the list is endless.

Possibly the worst offender is the modern 'vegetable oil'. Seemingly beneficial in name, these oils are often well known and have been used for centuries all over the world.

However, the food companies now refine these so that they do not spoil, using hydrogenation to extend the 'shelf-life' of supermarket and fast food products.

Firstly, the natural corn, sunflower, whatever oils are taken to very high temperatures and virtually all nutrition that was originally present in the seed or vegetable is lost. Worse, the refining process can use gasoline, ethylene, methylchloride and chlorination leaving behind chemical traces. Finally, in many cases the resulting liquid is fully or partially hydrogenated – they add hydrogen to make it more solid at room temperatures. This may be reheated and then pressed to make what you or I may think are healthy 'vegetable oil' margarines. A wolf in sheep's clothing.

Before the food companies got their chemical sets out, the main source of 'bad' fats was **saturated fats** – animal fats in meat, eggs, cheese and dairy. Excess, saturated fats are difficult to metabolise, they merely accumulate leading to a narrowing of the arteries and they are linked to increased cancer rates.

When oils are hydrogenated they are termed **trans fats**. For a number of years, people thought that the refining process just took out all the goodness and you were left with some sort of inert, nutritionally worthless oil. Not so. The Mayo Clinic comments, "A recent study of 80,000 nurses showed that women whose diets were high in both saturated and trans fats had an increased risk of heart attack. But of greater interest was the finding that nurses who consumed considerable amounts of trans fat faced an ever higher heart attack risk than nurses who ate a lot of saturated fat."

Ooooops!!

The Mayo Report continued, "The research adds to previous evidence that trans fat may be as bad for your heart as saturated fat. In fact, trans fat may even be more damaging because in addition to raising your 'bad' (LDL) cholesterol level, it also appears to lower your 'good' (HDL) cholesterol level."

We'll come to good and bad cholesterol later – let's not get confused!!

The New England Journal of Medicine has already gone further. In April 2006 a review entitled 'Trans fatty acids and Cardiovascular Disease' surely ended the debate. 'Trans fats are worse than saturated animal fats'. There is even research showing that trans fats stop you properly excreting waste.

So you can't win. If you don't want to plaster butter all over your toast because it is animal fat, you may turn to one of those healthy margarines with the picture of sunflowers all over the front. And that could well be worse!

The end product of the digestion of trans fats, just as with smoking, is free radicals. Lots of free radicals. As we said earlier, these molecules are incomplete; they have a missing piece and are quite happy to rip the replacement from any molecule they come across, in turn making this molecule incomplete. This in turn, rips pieces off other molecules until it is the genetic code that is being attacked, or the messages it directs inside the cell. And that increases your risk of cancer – enormously.

On top of all this, was the further finding in several research studies that both these trans fats and saturated fats can be converted in the body to **Prostaglandins**. There are predominantly three type of prostaglandin: PG1, PG2, and PG3. Saturated and trans fats have been proven to raise levels of PG2. Prostaglandins are just a few of about 130 local, cellular hormones called eicosanoids – and I will cover this in more detail in Chapter 20. In small amounts prostaglandins can be helpful. But large concentrations **they cause inflammation** and localised inflammation can be a precursor to, and a stimulus for, cancer.

In the USA trans fats have been named and shamed since January 2007. Products have to state their trans fat levels on pack and people now, rightly, steer clear of those which contain such fats. There has been a huge rush to clear trans fats from certain products – some fast food companies using 'No Trans Fats' as a marketing claim.

In Thailand I can find stickers stating the level of trans fats contained in my foods – why can't we in the UK? You really should do everything in your power to avoid these dangerous hydrogenated and trans fats.

Unsaturated fats

Finally, we have **'unsaturated'** fats – although even this category is not 'straightforward' to understand. Again, let me try to simplify it.

There are two main types of unsaturated fats:

- *Polyunsaturated fats*
  Polyunsaturated 'fats' are liquid at room temperature and are essential because the body cannot make them. Many margarines were launched on a healthier-for-you platform because they originated from these polyunsaturated oils. The list includes soybean, sunflower and safflower oils.

  But again, you must be very sure they haven't been through the processing and refining mill. And anyway, cooking with them obviously raises their temperature and starts to damage them.

  Linoleic acid is another important polyunsaturated oil. Found in vegetable oils, nuts, and seeds, this fat is important for growth and development as well as the production of hormone-like substances that regulate blood pressure.

  Polyunsaturated oils should provide around 2 per cent of your calories. In excess they can inhibit HDL levels (good cholesterol – see later) and also render vitamins like beta-carotene inert.

- *Monounsaturated fats*
  The 'healthiest' oils are monounsaturated oils found in, for example, **olive and walnut oils.** Bottles of pressed oils like these are easy to find around the Mediterranean and olive oil, in particular, has a high unsaturated, good fat content plus added benefits like polyphenols, and a number of research studies have linked its consumption with a decreased cancer risk.

  Ideally, you should choose bottles of these oils from a known supplier and in an untreated state. Oils high in monounsaturates are better for cooking as they have a high oxidation threshold and they remain stable on heating – so they do not become hydrogenated or saturated easily. Figures for the percentage of monounsaturated fat in nuts and seeds and oil are:

Olive oil	73%
Rapeseed oil	60%
Hazelnut	50%
Almonds	35%
Cashews	28%
Brazils	26%
Sesame seeds	20%
Pumpkin seeds	16%

But you still need to be careful of misleading claims for margarines containing them. The content could be minimal, and the margarine could be heavily refined and even hydrogenated.

Fish oils, flaxseed, linseed and other 'friendly' oils

There is another group of oils – a group I am going to call 'friendly oils'. Fish oils give you long-chain omega 3; whilst flaxseed, linseed and evening primrose give you predominantly short chain omega 3, omega 6 and a little omega 9. They are all essential oils, needed by our bodies.

I will cover this in more detail later, but suffice it to say here that you need as much long-chain omega 3 as you can get in this modern world, to balance the bad fats and to correct the over provision of omega 6 and 9 available in modern diets.

Omega 3 actually calms inflammation by switching off the enzymes that make prostaglandins.

So what have we learned from this?

You should observe some simple rules on your 'eat-to-beat cancer' diet.

- Ideally reduce total fat consumption to 10–20 per cent of total daily calorie intake.
- Eliminate all trans fats from your diet.
- Reduce consumption of saturated fats.
- Never eat fried food; especially out of home.
- Eat fresh whenever possible.
- Focus your oil and fat consumption on pure oils (e.g. olive, walnut), ideally from a source you can trust.
- Consume more oily fish, natural flaxseed and linseed

High cholesterol

High 'bad' cholesterol causes stagnation of the whole metabolic system and it specifically inhibits the ability of the liver to detoxify the blood and therefore the tissues. High cholesterol leads to more negative hormone production, especially oestrogen production and an increased risk of cancer.

High cholesterol may be caused for three reasons:

- You eat too much of it (the traditional medical view).
- You form too much of it in the body from other ingredients (the scientific evidence view).
- You fail to expel it via the liver.

Most people with 'high cholesterol' will be told to reduce their cholesterol intake (eggs, butter, lobster, shellfish, liver, cheese etc.) and that this will reduce their cholesterol levels in the body. This is tosh. The cholesterol molecule is far too large to cross the intestine wall. In other words, cholesterol is formed in the body from smaller molecules. And these can come from ingested fats, cholesterol and even carbohydrate! Hereditary factors can be important too.

Certain nutritional factors can help reduce your liver cholesterol levels: Magnesium, vitamins C, B-12 and B-6, plus lecithin
(choline, inositol, linoleic acid). As discussed earlier, people with
high cholesterol levels may well have bile duct blockages and
gallstones and should look seriously at undertaking a liver flush.

Also, you need to understand that there is cholesterol, and
there is cholesterol. HDL is the one you want; LDL is the one to
avoid. (High Density, rather than Low Density Lipoprotein.)
And a number of natural compounds switch the balance in
favour of the good one. Certain nutritional factors can reduce
your blood 'bad' cholesterol levels quite simply – like fish oils,
whole oat porridge, garlic, olive oil and taking probiotics.

- Having 2 per cent of your calorie intake as polyunsaturated
  oils reduce levels of LDLs, but above 10 per cent they inhibit
  the good guys, HDL's.
- The consumption of olive oil and other unsaturated fats is
  known to reduce the levels of bad LDL's, whilst leaving HDL's
  unaffected.
- Omega 3 has also been shown to reduce LDL's, as have plant
  fibres like lignans, and factors in whole oats do much the
  same.
- Having a healthy bacterial system in your gut has been shown
  in research studies, including clinical trials, to reduce the LDL
  levels. Certain beneficial bacteria can chop up foods to
  produce short chain esters and these reduce the formation and
  levels of LDL's.

Refined foods, processed foods and preserved foods

The food industry has a lot to answer for. Nowhere more so than
in its use of refining. Above we covered what they do when they
refine oils.

Grains: laughably, the food industry makes a virtue out of
foods being 'vitamin enriched' or having 'added fibre'. They
caused the problem in the first place. When they refine wheat, the
grain loses at least 75 per cent of its B vitamins, at least 90 per
cent of its mineral content, at least 98 per cent of its vitamin E
and at least 99 per cent of its fibre

You are eating pap. No wonder recent research in **icon** showed we are all becoming deficient in folate and several other B vitamins. This is costing lives and money: The NHS is even working with the drugs companies to perfect a 'Heart disease lowering pill' – one of its five ingredients is folic acid.

B vitamins like folic acid/folate are essential to the proper division and copying of our DNA.

Refined grains are used in processed foods and, along with chemicals, sugar and salt, E numbers and other additives; the consumer is getting little other than moderately toxic, nutritionally empty calories.

Ladies who lunch and go for their slimming plate of pasta and their glass of chardonnay are eating a food devoid of almost all its nutrition, where the refining process has actually increased the calorie level by about 7 per cent. Without a doubt, the glass of chardonnay provides more nourishment.

I have a simple rule – only put whole foods in your mouth.

Sadly, that won't solve all the problems with grains. The over-production and storage of grains in the EU has meant moulds are increasingly common, resulting in the presence of aflatoxin in the grains – and this is carcinogenic.

Meats and Meat Products: There is no requirement to label meats or meat products so the hormones, food additives, the drugs, antibiotics and chemicals used to fatten and treat the animal go unmentioned.

Nitrates are frequently added to brighten the meat. In fact sodium nitrite and nitrate are widely used in dried meats, bacon, pepperoni, sausages, hams and hot dogs. Children who consume more than a dozen hot dogs a month have a considerably higher (9.5 times) risk of leukaemia. Women eating these foods during pregnancy produce offspring with a higher incidence of brain cancer.

Pickling is linked to stomach and throat cancers (the Japanese eat a lot of pickled foods). Smoked meats and fish are also linked to stomach cancer.

But preservatives abound. In 1995 Americans each consumed on average ten pounds of preservatives. Britain is not far behind. Many different chemicals are used as preservatives, and yet no-one knows what effect this mix has on our bodies, and many of these chemicals may well have the ability to stay in our tissues for long periods of time.

A French police friend telling me about road accidents in France said that exhumed bodies were hardly decomposed two years after death, such was our exposure to chemical preservatives!

Sugar

Sugar abounds in our diets but is detrimental to our entire endocrine system. Increasingly nowadays people understand that they should try to avoid eating sugar wherever possible. The problem is sometimes people do not know it is there, or they don't realise just how much is there. Anything with an 'ose' (for example: fructose, sucrose) on the label is a sugar, and may be just a nutritionally deficient source of empty calories. For example, the ingredients of breakfast cereals, sucrose, corn sugar and honey, are still 'sugar'; in ketchup you have more sugar than is in ice cream, which anyway has a lot; fizzy soft drinks have up to 10 spoonfuls per can; 'healthy' Ribena has even more, and so on.

Sugar also significantly weakens your immune system. So called 'Healthy Fruit Smoothies' are laden with sugar and depress the immune system for 40 minutes to one hour after consumption.

Caffeine

Caffeine depletes the body of vitamins, especially B vitamins, essential for the correct division of cells. It is a poison and has a negative effect on the immune system and on potassium and magnesium levels. Recent research showed that taking paracetamol with coffee could cause liver damage.

Sweeteners

Saccharin for a while was linked to ovarian cancer, but was recently cleared. **Aspartame** is being studied by SDRT, the UK brain tumour charity, for possible links to child brain tumours. European research questioned its links to an increased risk of cancer, but the EU cleared it. However, in the USA, the Cancer Prevention Coalition has already pronounced against Aspartame.

In America brain tumours have recently overtaken leukaemia as the most common cancer in children.

Aspartame is in more than 5,000 food and drink items – from diet drinks to low fat yoghurts. It was originally developed as an ulcer medication but the FDA refused it a licence, deeming it unsafe for human consumption (FDA Public Board of Inquiry, Sept 30, 1980). Now permitted as a food additive, aspartame is a mix of six chemicals such as methanol, a cumulative poison known to affect sight. Methanol can also be converted under certain conditions to formaldehyde, a known carcinogen. Other ingredients include phenylalanine (linked to problems of the nervous system), and diketopiperazine, which has been demonstrated to cause brain tumours in animals.

Monosodium Glutamate

A totally unnecessary chemical food additive and flavour enhancer. It was developed by a food chemist in Japan. Early studies showed that it was addictive and could put weight on rats. John E. Erb wrote in his book 'The Slow Poisoning of America', that the whole purpose of adding MSG to food is to encourage people to eat more by enhancing taste. No legal limits have been set for the additive although it can cause a 'morning after' hangover, nausea, chest pains and numbness. Yummy.

Acrylamides

Panic set in early in 2002 when a Swedish scientist looking at whether toxins might be passing from plastic packaging into foods instead discovered highly toxic acrylamides present in chips (especially overly cooked ones), crisps and potato-bagged snacks, branded breakfast cereals, biscuits, crispbreads and crackers. Seemingly any oven-baked processed food where the temperature was taken over 120°c was liable to be contaminated.

The World Health Organisation says that the safe limit for acrylamides is zero, such is their concern. They immediately called together 26 of the world's top scientists to develop a viewpoint and some 'solutions'. Despite the severity of the findings no hard action has yet been taken – six years later! A study announced in January 2003 by Cancer Research UK attempted to say that the levels found in these foods were not found to cause 'long term' problems. Readers are nevertheless encouraged to exert caution as the findings came from a study lasting barely three months!

Indeed, in 2008 research from the University of Maastricht scientists analysing the eating habits of 120,000 people showed those who ate chips or crisps regularly were significantly more at risk of cancer.

For those concerned about acrylamides, three eat-to-beat cancer tips are:

- If you like to **snack,** make your own – put out a bowl of organic sunflower, pumpkin and sesame seeds, with a few chopped nuts.
- If you want a genuinely healthy **breakfast cereal** make your own with oats (unrefined), millet, chopped nuts, dried fruits, seeds, a little soya milk, rice milk or even water. Or eat organic whole oats – porridge made with water – and sprinkle some linseeds on top.
- Never roast quickly at high temperatures, only slowly at lower ones.

Eating 'out of home'

This may seem an odd inclusion, but not after you have given it some thought.

Some fast food chains only fry their food; some chains only microwave all their meals. Many restaurants will keep certain meats and fish in the freezer and microwave it to defrost it and avoid wastage.

Microwaved food is genetically modified food. When a microwave heats food it does it by exciting the electrons in the atoms of molecules. When the microwave is turned off do you think the electrons will all be in their original orbits? Kirlian photographs show microwaved food denuded of its natural energy and William Kopp has gathered together extensive German and Russian research. This shows that microwaved food is nutritionally deficient, and the number of cancer and pre-cancer cells circulating in the bloodstream rises after a microwaved meal.

Far Eastern food is little better. The Chinese food in the UK is often greasy and oily with monosodium glutamate and sugar widely used. You can get 6–12 gms of salt from one meal! Much of the dish Pad Thai is carbohydrate and oil in the UK complete with added sugar and nothing like the meal in Thailand.

The majority of restaurants use mass produced ingredients, and only those 'freshly' supplied by the supermarket down the road! Refined pasta, sugar and salt and dairy-laden sauces abound. It's a minefield for someone concerned about the quality of what they put into their body.

Summary

Above I have detailed some of the factors that could cut out perhaps 80 per cent of potential problems. But in all cases, I have tried to avoid the negative – providing simple ideas and alternatives you can use, from bowls of nuts and seeds, to olive oil, to taking probiotics, to eating whole grains, and whole oats – all of which can help you reduce the levels of free-radicals and cancer-feeding and cancer-producing agents in your body.

It's really not that hard, is it?

CHAPTER 14

ORGANIC FOOD – LIVING FOOD

Organic food really is better for you

There has been all too much mythology, false claim and counter claim about organic food. The debate is now over. Organic food really is better for you.

Various small studies have been trumpeted by the UK Soil Association over recent years. But now the arguments must surely cease. The EU has commissioned the definitive, £12 million study, growing organic crops and comparing them with mass-produced ones in several locations. (Quality Low Input Food, or the QLIF study). With the first results in, Professor Carlo Leifert (a patron of CANCERactive) and his team leading the study are quite clear: Organically produced crops and dairy milk usually contain far more 'beneficial compounds', like vitamins, minerals, omega 3 and antioxidants. More detailed results are expected over the next few years as the study continues.

We did know already. Over the last seven or eight years there have been some very serious and detailed studies done using matched research samples. What has become increasingly clear is that there are small increased levels of minerals in organic food, bigger increases in vitamins, but the biggest differences come when looking at certain important plant natural compounds like phenols, anthocyanins and so on. Not just inhibited by pesticides and herbicides, often the nitrogen-rich fertilisers get in the way of the plant producing these key, health providing factors. Here are just a few examples:

- Organic practices increase vitamin C levels in potatoes (Hajslova 2005).
- And strawberries (Asami 2003).
- Beta carotene levels are higher in organic crops (Lombardi-Boccia 2004).
- And high nitrogen fertilisers depress levels (Leclerc et al 1991).
- Plums grown organically with a ground cover of clover have

more polyphenols and quercitin (Lombardi-Boccia 2004).

- Organic potatoes and apples have higher levels of polyphenols and flavenols (Harmouz 1999).
- Organic strawberries have significantly higher levels of glutathione (Wang and Lin 2003).
- Resveratrol is 26 per cent higher in organic grapes.
- Phenolics are 33 per cent higher in organic peaches.
- Antioxidants are 220 per cent higher in organic spinach (Ren et al 2001).
- Chinese cabbage and Welsh onions have 1.3 to 10.4 times the anti-mutagenic flavenoid concentrations (Ren 2001).

Is your food organic?

What really is organic food? My definition would be that it is a natural food, grown in its fully natural state, in balance with its natural environment. Crop rotation plays an important part in my definition. For example, it allows nitrogen fixing bacteria to play their role and different crops to recharge the soil to the benefit of the next crop.

Our bodies and our DNA have evolved to be in balance with the world around us over hundreds of thousands of years. It was a slow steady process of development. Most of us are wise enough to realise that pouring chemicals into our environment suddenly leaves our bodies unprepared to meet the sudden changes. So too with food.

But, since the ancient Egyptians, we have always strived to create bigger chickens, potatoes that avoided the blight or new crops that grew even with low rainfall. When we cross-bred two potatoes in the eighteenth century, was the resultant potato natural? When we cross-bred wild turkeys to create the domestic version, or two breeds of chicken to make a better egg-layers, are our bodies ready? Or seedless grapes and oranges, are they truly natural?

But now 'cross-breeding' has reached new levels. Led by American food company scientists we now 'play' with the natural DNA freely producing 'genetically modified seeds'. Approximately 99 per cent of the GM seeds now used are of two types – about 79 per cent is herbicide-resistant, and 20 per cent is pesticide-producing. The claimed benefit is that the volumes of crops produced per acre will grow, and that ultimately we will need less herbicides and pesticides in our fields. The reality is that the level of these chemical toxins required does not seem to have declined by the fifth year and herbicide resistant weeds are now on the increase. And every year farmers, however poor, need to buy new seed instead of gathering their own because these special GM seeds, uniquely, have been allowed to be patented by the US Government. The farmer even has to contract to buy the herbicide solely from the seed company too.

Critics claim that the process of genetic modification can generate other potentially dangerous genetic fragments within the seed. They are concerned that the seed companies have been allowed to write their own rules, the FDA granting them virtual self regulation. There also seems to be insufficient testing, especially for potential side effects.

The French, for example, have resisted American companies' suggestions to grow genetically modified crops. And the decision seems to be supported by the facts. There are already studies showing increased cancer risks from GM potatoes (Institute of Nutrition of the Russian Academy, 1998) and several others using potatoes, corn, soy and canola have shown liver damage in animals, while others have shown that GM fed animals had impaired gene expression, greater mortality and more organ damage overall. Smaller babies are also observed. In other cases (for example with GM Soy) higher incidence of allergies is noted.

Perhaps most alarming is an observation by Judy Carman an Epidemiologist and GM expert, when reviewing Food Standards Australia New Zealand conclusions about the safety of GM foods, that they overlooked potential problems including birth defects, cancer and long-term nutritional deficiencies. '*A review of 12 feeding trials includes none with people, and one where the seed was not even tested with animals*'. Tests usually only monitored effects after 7 to 14 days and then only looked for any effects from the planned genetic change and not for any side effects or unplanned effects. Some experiments only tested the foods with five or six animals.

More concerns are emerging over crops with genetic

mutations designed to resist bacteria; could they have a detrimental effect on the beneficial bacteria in your intestine? The FDA has actually prepared a report on the fear that Antibiotic Resistant Marker genes (ARM) could transfer into the beneficial bacteria of the intestine. One FDA report actually wrote in capital letters that ARM would be a SERIOUS HEALTH HAZARD as they could create a new breed of bacteria immune to antibiotics.

Bizarrely, the French are looking seriously at allowing one crop to 'go' GM: Grapes! Between 1999 and 2005 there have been 25 tests on GM grapes in America. And the French have been working on GM grapes with the Italians Germans and Australians. GM strains for herbicide resistance and mould resistance have been developed; one even helps the grapes to resist mould by producing hydrogen cyanide! As you will understand later, the development of mould on the skins of organic grapes actually causes the grape to produce resveratrol, which we are only just learning is a highly important natural compound in the fight against cancer and a number of other diseases like Alzheimer's. And it is the very compound that gives the grape, and red wine its image of health.

Seven out of every ten supermarket foods in the USA now contain GM strains.

And how can a judge decide that it is 'safe' to have a GM crop 60 yards or 80 yards from a natural one? Birds eat seeds, they fly, they deposit the seeds miles away and the next year the pollen interacts with a natural crop. Is our evolution really to be left to ageing judges with no knowledge of science and Darwinian principles?

One estimate I read stated that there could be no natural crops in the USA in five years time. Is that what we want in Europe?

Even Organic food is not beyond political influence: The demand for organic food has grown dramatically in both the US and the UK. The two countries have had rather different solutions. In the US the solution was merely to change the rules and regulations, bringing with it concerns that the food could not be trusted to be truly organic. By contrast the Brits kept the stringent rules in place and import foods to make up the shortfall. Let us hope that the Soil Association has world-wide policing of Kenyan green bean crops and Vietnamese mangoes. Why am I so concerned?

Mass production

The sad truth is that when it comes to food we continually confuse quantity with quality, volume with value, eating with nourishment.

One example of this is the emergence of 'Hydrophonic farming'. By 2010 there will be a complex in Kent the size of ten soccer pitches growing 1.3 million tomato, pepper and cucumber plants all year round, using no soil, but a liquid solution instead. Current estimates are that this one 'factory' will produce 15 per cent of the UK's salad crop production – reducing reliance on imports. While natural predators not pesticides will control pests enhancing the 'organic' image of the end product, the 'food' will be grown on rock wool – rock that has had air blown through it and resembles candy floss – in a solution of water, nitrogen, phosphate, potassium and magnesium. If the tomatoes are receiving no trace minerals, how will you? The debate has started in the press, but it is one of overcoming food shortages versus loss of food taste. Does anyone think about nourishing your cells anymore? Has anyone conducted any proper research on vitamin, mineral and natural compound content of these all year round crops against the natural, organic varieties of our forefathers?

But producing more lettuces unnaturally is really the tip of the iceberg. There are a number of basic reasons to be concerned about mass-market, supermarket crops. Firstly, fields are repeatedly sown with the same crop. the idea of crop rotation seems to have died in the Middle Ages. Of course there was reason to it. Crop rotation was used to recharge depleted soils with certain bacteria and nutrients across the 4 year cycle. Now chemical fertilisers are expected to do the job just as well. Unfortunately they don't and they can't. Take the loss of minerals for example. One study using the UK Government' own figures over a 50 year period to 1990 showed losses of minerals like calcium in green vegetables reaching 70 per cent, and another showed vitamin E declines to merely one sixth of the levels 100 years ago. How could synthetic fertilisers be expected to make up these shortfalls in fields planted with the same crops each year?

Furthermore, in the attempt to sell more premium products, or simply to keep their shelves fully stocked, supermarkets seek more produce from abroad. But vitamin levels are all about the ripening process of the vegetable or fruit. And they are lost quite quickly in stored fruit and vegetables. Within four or five days of picking, most green vegetables have lost 50 per cent of their vitamins and a potato has lost three quarters of its vitamin C (and potatoes are the UK's best natural home-grown source of the vitamin). By the time the produce has reached the UK, been unloaded, shipped to a central storage location and then out to the supermarkets, what nourishment can we expect to have left?

Frozen vegetables fare little better with 25 to 50 per cent of the vitamins disappearing upon freezing.

Minerals are absorbed from the soil throughout the full development of the fruit. Pick the food after only 60 or 70 per cent of its full growth span and expect the consequences.

How could we ever expect the same vitamin and mineral content in supermarket produce as in 'Locally grown fruits and vegetables, in season and picked ripe and eaten fresh'? Macrobiotic principles don't seem that absurd at all.

But it is not simply a question of vitamins and minerals. I have Kirlian photographs of mass market foods and their organic equivalents, and they show clearly that organic food has more 'energy' in it than non-organic. To repeat: Food is supposed to nourish my body and provide it with vitality. How will eating lifeless, energy-less, vitamin and mineral reduced foods do this?

Pesticides and herbicides

Another benefit of organic foods is that they should contain no pesticides or herbicides; no toxins to weaken our immune systems or damage the balance of hormones inside our bodies. With 'normal' vegetables and fruit there is little legislation restricting what pesticides and insecticides are used, nor how often. Over 400 fertilisers, herbicides and pesticides are available for use on our farms. Is it any wonder that farmers have a higher incidence of multiple myeloma and leukaemia?

Pesticides and insecticides have also been linked with brain tumours, connective tissue tumours (especially with children), and liver cancer and are thought to be behind the recent rapid growth of kidney cancer. Whilst individual pesticides might be found in any food at a level lower than the Government's desig?nated safe level, the Government has done little research on the interaction of all the chemicals, or indeed the cumulative and interactive build up over a number of years within the tissues of the human body.

In the USA, the lifetime maximum safe limit set for these chemicals is exceeded when a baby reaches the age of 18 months!

Fruit orchards can be sprayed a dozen times, then the fruit is waxed locking the pesticide in. Long gone are the days when chickens populated orchards to eat the bugs before the bugs could climb the trees!

Worse, for example, when Western governments banned DDT, they only banned its use. Some unscrupulous companies are still free to sell these chemicals to third world buyers. And do you know where your green beans and lettuce were actually grown? The Food Standards Agency in the UK stated in 2006 that increasingly certain imported foods contain higher levels of pesticides than is legally deemed safe. But do we actually ban their sale?

Worry about the bees

Albert Einstein once said that if all the bees died out man would only live another four years. This could be prophetic. The issue facing world leaders is not the price of oil and food, but the loss of bees. They are dying out. Various theories have suggested pesticides, GM crops, EMF's from masts and mites, cuckoo-like bugs that get inside the hive and lay their eggs inside the bee brood cells, stunting the growth of the next generation of bees. Flowers, most vegetables, virtually all fruit (except bananas), clover and wild herbs would all die out. And that also means great reductions for cotton, feed for cattle and even precursors for herbal medicines and drugs. Olive oil, nuts, grains like corn and oats, and rice would still be with us – they don't need pollination. The Armageddon scenario has actually started. In some regions farmers are pollinating orchards by hand. Whatever the cause, someone in power needs to come up with some answers soon. Meanwhile, since there is not a lot you and I can do about this, let's keep going with our current plans to improve our nourishment:

Saving money while going organic

But 'going organic' is not an option for everybody because of the increased expense. The good news is that not all contaminated foods were created equal! According to the Environmental Working Group of Washington DC, people can lower their pesticide exposure by 90 per cent by choosing their fruits and vegetables wisely. Eating the 12 most contaminated fruits and vegetables will expose a person to nearly 20 pesticides each day, says the EWG. So they are the ones to buy in organic versions. At the other end of the spectrum there are foods which are sprayed little and/or absorb little. If you just want to avoid the chemicals you might as well buy the supermarket versions. For your information, they have now completed three studies and the findings have been consistent, with fruits worse than vegetables.

12 most contaminated		*12 least contaminated*	
Apples	Peaches	Asparagus	Mangoes
Red bell peppers	Pears	Avocados	Onions
Celery	Potatoes	Bananas	Papaya
Cherries	Red Raspberries	Broccoli	Pineapples
Grapes	Spinach	Cauliflower	Peas
Nectarines	Strawberries	Kiwi	Sweetcorn

A 2000 Study by the Consumer Union reflected the same pollution. Apples, peaches, pears, grapes, green beans, spinach, strawberries and watermelon were the foods with the highest levels of pesticide residues.

However, it may not be hard to put matters right. Another group of scientists, this time the Centre for Disease Control and Prevention at the University of Washington, funded by the US Government, tested the urine samples of school children in Seattle for 'organophosphate pesticides'. During a 15 day trial, those consuming organic foods saw their levels drop to zero.

Meat and fish

Nearly 60 per cent of the calories we consume from processed animal products (for example meats, dairy, cheese, etc.) come from fat. As we said earlier, fat is a wonderful solvent and contains toxic chemicals and antibiotics from the upbringing and diet of the animal. Over one hundred such substances have been identified and 40 per cent of them are carcinogenic.

In the USA 82 drugs, hormones and chemicals are legally allowed to be given to dairy herds. Growth hormone and oestrogen are two of these and one has to accept that any meat consumption comes with these chemicals contained in the flesh and especially the fat. Dairy consumption brings a similar chemical concoction.

Then there are the antibiotics, colourings and, depending upon the previous crops in the fields where they graze, possibly high levels of pesticides and insecticides from the fields. The foodstuffs may not even be natural. BSE in cattle was brought about by feeding animal food products to herbivores. Whatever happened to the concept of animal husbandry?

Farmed fish often do not consume the sorts of food they would have eaten in their natural habitat. Natural plankton is essential for their omega 3 levels, but will hardly be found in the waters of farms. Farmed fish also have 20 per cent more 'fat' than their wild ancestors due to their own 'sedentary' existence!

The mass market animals have weakened immune systems and are more prone to parasites, bacteria and viruses. The incidence of liver fluke in British livestock has increased four-fold since 1997. Recently Asian prawns and chickens, which had been banned for consumption by humans because of toxins, were found to have been shipped for use by EU farmers as animal food! The toxins entered the food chain nevertheless! Volume and profit margins have become the Holy Grails of food creation. Nourishment is an old-fashioned concept.

Action?

• Eat-to-beat cancer means that you should take more trouble over selecting the products that go into your mouth. Know a few reliable suppliers. And buy locally-grown, fresh, in season and organic where possible. Shop more often if necessary.

- Why not start your own vegetable garden and plant a few fruit trees? You will be surprised how easy they are to grow along the fence instead of those leylandii.

CHAPTER 15

DERIVING THE MAXIMUM NOURISHMENT FROM YOUR DIET

Say 'beneficial bacteria' to most doctors and they just might mention something about little milky drinks with more than an added hint of marketing.

But the truth is somewhat different. In the last 7 years we have seen a huge scientific breakthrough in our understanding of the role and crucial importance of beneficial bacteria to the body's health systems. In fact there has been an explosion in our understanding, and I don't blame your doctor or oncologist if he is simply not up to speed with it all. Over 1000 research studies and 80 clinical trials have taken place in the last 5 years alone on this very 'hot' topic.

The secret source of your good health

Beneficial bacteria have **five important roles** in your intestines:

- They are the first line of your immune defenses. At night when you sleep, they attack and digest most of the microbes and yeasts you ingested during the day – ones you would rather not have in your body at all.
- And, what is becoming increasingly clear is that they are not just the front line foot soldiers, they actually direct the formation of about 80 per cent of all your immune defences throughout your body!
- They work with your digestive system to extract certain important natural compounds from your foods – like vitamin K, B-12, folic acid and more. Without them you just cannot derive full nourishment from your foods.
- They also produce some unique natural compounds from your foods which can promote better health.
- They can chelate to (bind with) toxins – like oestrogen, nitrosamines and heavy metals, using certain natural compounds in fibrous foods to help expel them from your body.

129

The prime cause for concern is that, with the exception of a few UK professors waving warning flags, the Government Health programme, the Orthodox Medical Community and the drugs companies are just killing them off willy-nilly with little regard for their importance.

The facts

Over 800 different types of bacteria live in your gut. About 400 have been identified, and a dozen or so commonly feature in much of the latest research. These include:

- Lactobacillus Bulgaris, Acidophilus, Shirota, Caseii. Lactis, Rhamnosus, Plantarum
- Bifidobacterium bifidum
- Streptocococcus thermohilus, and
- Saccharomyces boulardi

By 'infecting' us, bacteria such as these produce an immune response and stimulate our immune system into action. Research shows that these 'friendly bacteria' direct our defences. They increase the numbers of T- and B-lymphocytes, immunoglobulins, cytokines and Natural Killer cells in our bodies. Rather like certain vaccines, they help 'immunise' us against a worse attack that might come in the future. Without them your immune system withers, and is simply less prepared to face a major threat if and when one occurs.

Research over recent years has linked a lack of beneficial bacteria to all manner of illnesses from allergies like asthma to heart disease and cancer. If you don't have a wide range of happy and well fed bacteria in your gut you will not have a strong immune system. It is as simple as that,

Breaking the relationship that protects us

One hundred years ago when we lived on farms, we all ate a bit of dirt daily. Hands that touched chickens, horses and dogs then fed the babies. We constantly ate bacteria from a variety of sources. Importantly these could have included some not-so-common strains. For example, when young children 'pick up colds' it may just be that they are reacting to a new bacterial strain that has entered their system. Research studies show that children brought up on farms, and children brought up in homes that have animals have much stronger immune systems. For life!

Natural birth babies have much stronger immune systems too – they pick up bacteria passing through the birth canal. Mother's breast milk contains specific polysaccharides that feed certain beneficial bacteria in baby, increasing their immune system. Bottled milk doesn't. And so on.

Now our rapidly changing, sanitised world that is no longer rural but sees 72 per cent of us living in towns and cities, offers surgical not natural birth, and pasteurises, sterilises, irradiates and cleans fastidiously means that we just don't eat these guys in the volumes we used to.

Worse, we actually kill them off. With prescribed antibiotics and drugs, chemotherapy and mercury-based vaccines, but also with everyday factors like chlorinated water, or antibiotics in our food, or too much salt which changes the acidity of our digestive juices to a point where the bacteria don't like swimming in it. Our friendly bugs can be wiped out in unfriendly conditions in just three days.

And when we kill them off, some of them are not so easy to replace – the bacterium you ingested from the cat when you were four years old is only found occasionally. All that immune response and protection may be lost forever.

Finally, we also no longer give them the foods they enjoy, like whole foods, vegetables and importantly fibre and so we break our deal with them. And it's a deal that has built up over several million years. You look after me – and I'll look after you. It is called symbiosis.

Optimising your body against cancer

So, in summary, I'd like to put this very clearly and simply: If you don't have the right strains of beneficial bacteria in your gut, and in the right numbers, you will find it virtually impossible to beat cancer. Beneficial bacteria are a crucial part of your defence system. They:

- Digest the invading microbes and particularly yeasts that could cause you problems.
- Direct and strengthen your immune system – developing extra white cells that can better identify, attack and digest cancer cells.

Next they combine with the digestive juices to cut up your food for you. They do this with whole fibrous foods – they simply cannot help you, if you don't help them. Fed properly, research shows that:

- They release vitamin K from your greens – important in protecting the liver against metastasis.
- They 'produce' B vitamins like biotin, folic acid and B-12 – important in the copying process, and in repairing DNA and even killing cancer cells.
- They produce short chain esters from certain carbohydrates. Once in the blood stream these reduce 'bad' cholesterol levels – important in reducing bad fat levels and eliminating toxins.

Next, they help you remove harmful and toxic waste from your body.

- They bind to and help excrete certain heavy metals like cadmium and mercury
- They bind to oestrogenic products – human and chemical
- They bind to nitrosamine compounds – which can increase the risks of certain cancers, like colorectal

An example: Colon cancer

Various research studies on colon cancer show that it is linked to low B-12 and folic acid levels, inflammation, nitrosamines from burnt meats and localised oestrogen, and risk doubles if you double your salt intake. Washington University and Tokyo have shown that the potential metastatic secondary, liver cancer, can be halted by vitamin K supplementation.

I have long held that the cause of colon cancer and the most often metastasis – to the liver – was actually microbes or parasites. In 2007 American research showed exactly that. And if microbial infection predominates it is because you no longer have the right balance, conditions and foods to provide for a healthy intestinal flora that could defeat the microbe. All the factors research has shown are associated with colon cancer are in fact factors associated with a lack of beneficial bacteria.

Eat-to-beat cancer

Clearly the start point is to avoid chlorinated tap water, and mass market meats with added antibiotics. You might also decide you should avoid drugs, salt, and especially antibiotics. Then there is a simple rule – only put food in your mouth that is 'whole' – food which contains lots of natural fibre. So avoid mass market packaged and processed foods, and refined sugars and carbohydrates – this is not part of the deal you have made with these friendly guests.

If you can't live on a farm, it is essential that you 'top up' with as many strains of beneficial bacteria as you can get each day – five to ten different ones would be the minimum. The way to do this is to take a probiotic. A probiotic cannot be called a probiotic unless it has been shown in clinical trials that the beneficial bacteria in the bottle can reach their desired destination (the way through the stomach is paved with acidic danger) and, once there, they can deliver a clear, proven health benefit. Yakult gives you Shirota; Prebiota 7 and Neways Advanced Probiotic give you 7 and 6 different strains respectively. Always take the pills with cold water.

Then you need to feed them correctly. Certain beneficial bacteria like certain foods (called prebiotics). Mother's milk will stimulate *bifidobacterium*; inulin in onions and chicory will stimulate *L. acidophilus*. Whole, fresh, natural foods please. They don't like junk food, they are very picky eaters.

This is a very serious subject. Your oncologists and doctors won't know about it, the drugs companies don't want to even acknowledge it. But if you want to beat cancer you need a healthy intestinal flora to give you the best immune system possible, and nutrients that can help fight and beat the disease. When eminent professors say that changing your diet doesn't matter a jot, I wonder if all the patients in the research had taken the usual list of antibiotics, steroids and chemotherapy drugs. No wonder the foods didn't help. The patients' bodies couldn't derive any nourishment from them; their immune system had no stimulus!

CHAPTER 16
VITAMINS AND MINERALS IN THE FIGHT AGAINST CANCER

If you ever need an example of people being seriously confused, you need look no further that the Medical Community and their understanding of 'Vitamin Supplements'. Increasingly they class these as part of 'CAM' – Complementary and Alternative Medicine. Note the word 'medicine'. It means they want to regulate vitamin supplements just as they think they do drugs!

Before we get into the detail of this section I want to make my views clear up front – they are all based on scientific research.

1. **Nothing is better for you that eating the actual food or full natural compound.** For example, research scientists gave identical matched samples of people, identical doses of vitamin C from synthetic tablet or fresh orange juice. At intervals between 3 and 24 hours later, blood samples from each group were stressed with hydrogen peroxide, and oxidative damage measured. The blood samples that had come from the orange juice takers, resisted the damage quite significantly. The samples where the pills had been taken had no effect. Researchers felt that the reason for the difference was that orange juice had a combination of advantageous factors over and above vitamin C, like flavones, carotenoids and cyanidin-3-glucoside plus the natural sugars to enhance the effect. (Guarnieri; British Journal of Nutrition 2007; 97).

2. **Chemically synthesised supplements may even be dangerous.** There have been several meta-studies from the USA, the Cochrane Institute and others – all claiming that antioxidants like beta-carotene and vitamin E could reduce life expectancy. Importantly, while researchers laid themselves open to criticism by actively selecting less than 10 per cent of possible studies available (causing bodies like Cancer Research UK to question the objectivity), the

research studies chosen largely involved synthetic compounds and not natural vitamins, which nobody seems to have picked up on!

3. **Natural compounds that help beat cancer extend way beyond a few common antioxidants.** There is an ongoing myopia that 'vitamin supplements' are synonymous with 'antioxidants' and usually this means vitamins C, E and beta-carotene. These are only a very small proportion of the compounds that might help a cancer patient. There is a great deal of new research on a variety of natural compounds – from vitamins like K and D, to whole compounds like fish oils, curcumin, ellagic acid, quercitin and resveratrol. Many of these compounds when taken from natural sources with their associated co-factors are proving extremely useful in the fight against cancer.

4. **Mineral supplementation is becoming increasingly essential.** While minerals such as selenium and zinc are commonly quoted as essential to the anti-cancer process, other minerals, especially trace minerals like boron, are now being found to play important roles too. But as I am showing, whether due to mass production farming, soil depletion and lack of crop rotation, or hydrophonic growing methods, mineral levels are in serious decline in our everyday foods.

Toxicity and nutritional deficiency

Earlier in the book I explained that when I talk to, or correspond with, newly diagnosed cancer patients it takes but a very short while to find proof that they are both toxic and nutritionally deficient – leading to a weakening of their immune systems and the development of disease. **Toxicity** can be divided into two parts:

*   **Toxicity from external third party issues** – like chemicals, drugs, pesticides, EMF's etc. I believe I have shown that in many of these cases, there are effective ways of detoxing the body. By this I do not mean running off to the health food shop for a herbal drink. It is known that selenium will help displace heavy metals like mercury from the body; chlorella

has a similar ability to bind to such poisons, as do plant lignans and, as we will see, indole-3-carbinol in broccoli and greens is being developed and patented by pharmaceutical companies, such is its excellent abilities. All this is aided by the action of the correct beneficial bacteria in the gut. There is much research on this and even many clinical trials.

- **Toxicity due to a poor mineral imbalance** – again I believe I have covered the need to ensure you are a potassium- and magnesium-rich machine, not a sodium- and dairy calcium-rich one.

Nutritional deficiency is a product of our modern lifestyles, and the rubbish purporting to be food that surrounds us these days.

The Food Standards Agency in the UK has told us that, *'People do not need supplementation if they are eating a balanced diet.'* When we asked what a balanced diet was they told us that it was, *'Eating a bit of everything, with emphasis on starchy foods and 5 portions of fruit and vegetables a day'* (we have the letter).

Firstly, people like doctors and the FSA forget that the NHS actually recommends supplementation themselves – for example folic acid in certain cases like pregnancy and heart disease. Next, the Government is currently looking at a daily supplement to reduce heart disease – containing folic acid, a beta-blocker and a statin – for all people over 55 years of age. Finally, doctors regularly hand out supplements, but of synthetic hormones which are many, many times more potent than vitamins – HRT and thyroxin being but two examples. And what of the negative research on HRT? I've never seen studies on vitamin C that show it can cause more cancers, heart problems and even kill people.

Secondly, our modern lifestyles are not totally of our making but they can control our diets. For example, a businessman flying to Frankfurt for a day's meeting at 6.30 in the morning has little choice but to supplement. Modern no-frills airlines have only crisps, bagged snacks, and refined flour sandwiches to eat. A hastily taken sandwich often substitutes for lunch. Where is the nourishment in this? Surely a multi-vitamin and mineral supplement would be a good, if not essential, idea?

Finally, we have covered the poor diets of our children and their pizzas and crisps and chocolate. But if they turned to the staple foods in our supermarkets to *'eat a bit of everything including starchy foods'*, what would they find? Nutritionally worthless foods like refined rice and pasta, and white bread, and sugar. In some supermarkets you cannot find wholewheat pasta, or whole brown rice. The vegetables and fruit are not a lot better. Often picked unripe and shipped half way round the world – not exotic ones but potatoes, green beans and broccoli, raspberries and pears. Red peppers, tomatoes and lettuces grown in 'nourishing' liquids not soil, to shorten the growing time!

Vitamin and mineral depletion

Our soils are increasingly depleted. Crops are grown for volume and frequency, crop rotation is rarely used, natural seasons have been shortened, resulting in certain fields barely even rested as one crop of wheat follows another.

In February 2004 David Thomas, a mineralogist, published a paper investigating the decline of mineral levels in our fruits and vegetables from 1940 to 1990, using the government's own figures. The report showed major declines of up to 70 per cent in potassium, magnesium, iron and calcium. A second, separate study, by Anne-Marie Mayer of Cornell University was published in the *Bristol Food Journal* and made similar conclusions.

The US Senate minutes in 1936 stated that laboratory tests had proven that US farm soils were becoming minerally depleted, as was the produce, and that people were developing deficiencies. This was repeated in the senate hearing in 2002. The fact is that the FSA recommendation that you don't need supplementation is in complete contrast to US recommendations – there have been three senate hearings on the subject and the recommendation was that people should supplement, especially with minerals as the soils growing the crops were increasingly depleted.

But our weakened soils are only the start. Other factors reduce your vitamin and mineral intake and nourishment. To recap the various points I have made:

• Much of the produce we eat has travelled a long distance. It

may be a week between picking and eating, or more.
- Much of the produce we eat, especially fruit, has been picked unripe anyway so that it does not go off during the week of travel nor when on shelf in store.
- Fruits gain the majority of their vitamins as they ripen. Unripe fruit may be 50 to 60 per cent deficient.
- Broccoli, brassicas, spinach, asparagus lose 50 per cent of their vitamins within five days of picking. A potato will lose 75 per cent of its vitamin C within 5 days. Fruits can lose 50 per cent of their vitamin C within 1 day.
- Frozen vegetables lose about a third of their vitamins during the freezing process.

Also, the FSA can tell us that there is no need to supplement – but they don't seem to have studied the latest scientific research. For example, vitamin E depletion in vegetables like cabbage and lettuce has resulted in levels around one sixth of those found in 1900. If you look at the research being done on vitamin E and cancer, the scientists show that levels of 200 mgs (about 300 International Units or IU's) for vitamin E give results. If I started to eat vitamin E rich food when I woke up and carried on all day, I would be lucky to get past 100 IU's. Without supplementation how am I going to get to the levels scientists show are effective?

Then there are important compounds like Coenzyme Q10. As we age we make less of it, but it is vital to the perfect workings of our power stations, the mitochondria, and is used by Gonzalez and Gerson to fight cancer. The good news is that you can supplement. US research showed that supplementation of 30-50 mgs per day (any more is wasted) produces results after about 3 months and restores levels to those found in people in their mid-twenties. If we take the FSA route of eating a bit of everything to increase our levels, then you will need about 3 meals a day of brains, liver, kidney and other offal. Delicious – I think I'll take the supplements.

Do antioxidants work with cancer?

Let's start with simple antioxidants and multivitamins. Three very large real life studies show they do. These were not done in a laboratory, in a test tube or with mice. These were all real time studies with humans and matched samples.

- The US conducted a five-year study of 38,000 people in China, finishing in 1993. It showed that the group of people supplied daily with three antioxidants (beta-carotene, vitamin E and selenium) had a 13 per cent reduction in cancers, and a 21 per cent decline in death from cancer despite their already supposed healthy diets.
- The French completed the seven year Su. Vi. Max study in Autumn 2003. 17,000 people took a single pill containing 5 antioxidants (zinc, selenium, beta-carotene and vitamins E and C) in a random, blind test. During the research period there were 31 per cent less men's cancers and 37 per cent less cancer deaths overall.
- A 30 year diary study on eating habits in the USA on colon cancer showed that those people who took a multivitamin and mineral supplement in the 1970's and 80's at least 4 times per week went on to get 40 per cent less colon cancers.

The fact is that these supplements help prevent. And they help correct if you have it. And they help you survive. And they seem to work quite fast.

'New' vitamins

But, it is too easy to focus on 'the famous 5 antioxidants' as if they were the panacea for everything. Part of the reason is that doctors and press alike have just about understood that free radicals rush around in our bodies 'oxidising' things and so antioxidants are there to stop them. And so vitamin C, beta-carotene and vitamin E are pulled out of the cupboard again and again to be extolled or attacked, depending upon which day of the week this is.

This belittles the important scientific evidence being produced by researchers all over the world.

You will also find doctors and other health professionals – I even heard it from the CEO of a UK cancer charity – saying, *'There's just no evidence to support the use of supplements'*. If they believe that they are clearly very ignorant – apart from the above three studies, go to any US cancer web site – try Harvard Medical School, the Mayo Clinic, UCLA, MD Anderson; AND in the UK, www.canceractive.com and you will see just how ignorant! There you will find that:

- The EU approved form of vitamin E – synthetic alpha toco-pherol – is the form of least ability. The tocotrienol forms have considerable new research behind them (from the USA and Japan especially) on their cancer preventing effects. Indeed alpha-tocopherol may even block the action of tocotrienols.
- Vitamin D is seen by Harvard Medical School as essential in the fight against cancer – cancer cells actually have more vitamin D receptor sites than healthy cells and vitamin D kills them. Recommended Daily Allowances (RDA's) were set for the prevention of Rickets – the new research shows them woefully low.
- Vitamin K is now being shown by the Universities of Washington and Tokyo to be able to stop some cases of liver cancer and leukaemia. RDA's were originally set for blood clotting issues – again they are woefully low for cancer prevention.

Vitamin supplementation with orthodox therapies

Many patients go to their doctors asking if it is safe to carry on taking their supplements when he is giving them his orthodox concoctions of radio or chemotherapy. Since he doesn't actually know anything about supplements, but worries that his medicine anyway may fail, he will tell patients that they should stop taking the supplements as they can interfere with his clever stuff. He may say they are contra-indicated with the drugs or use other similar terms of 'Doctorspeak'. He will then probably add that they should just eat a healthy diet including five lots of fruit and vegetables a day. Clearly then he believes that a healthy diet is devoid of all vitamins and minerals that could possibly interfere in any way at all.

We have even had **icon** kicked out of hospitals because we dared to say that there is research showing certain vitamins and natural compounds can improve the success of radiotherapy. The oncologist in charge said we were irresponsible and said that our suggested supplements were contra-indicated. When we asked for his evidence to pass on to our readers, we received none at all. It simply doesn't exist. In fact, the opposite is true:

In 2001, John Boik of MD Anderson stated that Natural Compounds could actually enhance the effects of radio and chemotherapy. This was after he had reviewed over 4,000 scientific research studies for his book *'Natural Compounds in Cancer Therapy'*. This was also the conclusion of UCLA in 2004 who stated that whilst healthy cells controlled their uptake of antioxidants and 'stopped' when they'd enough, cancer cells had lost this control and antioxidants could move into a cancer cell in excess and help the radio or chemotherapy destroy it.

Ralph Moss has published a paper in PubMed, following a review of all the published evidence. In this review he reiterates that the case against taking vitamins during these orthodox therapies has no supporting research evidence.

Moreover, the truth is that **there are clinical trials that support the benefit of supplements with chemotherapy.** Here are just a few little examples:

- Tocotrienol vitamin E actually enhances the effects of Tamoxifen, so much so that you need 25 per cent less of the drug if you take the right dose of vitamin E in the right form. You won't hear too much about this research as far less Tamoxifen would be sold if women decided that they'd rather take some vitamin E and cut their risks of side-effects and womb cancer. There are also clinical studies on indole-3-carbinol a natural compound, which also reduces the volume of Tamoxifen required.
- MD Anderson in 2007 showed that both vitamin K3 and vitamin C improved the success rates of chemotherapy drugs in clinical trials in bladder cancer.
- Canadian researchers (British Journal of Cancer) showed that using fumaric acid, a natural compound, helped activate an enzyme which enhances the activity of a drug called mitomycin C, used against solid tumours in the bowel and bladder. The combination allowed the drug to be used at lower doses with less side effects.

- MD Anderson have also proven that resveratrol has a huge potential for fighting cancer and it can also improve the success rates of chemotherapy, appearing safe even in high doses.
- Other US cancer centers use vitamin D especially with breast cancer patients.
- The herb Uno de Gato (cat's claw) has been shown to protect healthy cells during chemotherapy, whilst having no interference with its action on cancer cells. It also boosts the immune system simultaneously.

And with radiotherapy:

- St Thomas' Hospital has some research (but no clinical trials as yet) to show that both isoflavones and selenium can improve the success of radiotherapy.
- MD Anderson repeated German research using astragalus to deliver enhanced radiotherapy results. They have found that it can double survival times.
- Harvard and others have used vitamin D with radiotherapy and shown improved outcomes.

Protection to nearby healthy cells, while minimising side effects like hair loss, can be helped by eating foods such as organic eggs, whole grains and greens for the organic iron and B vitamin (especially folic acid) content. Or you can supplement with B complex containing 400 mgs of folic acid. This has been proven to help reduce damage to the healthy cells.

Fish oils and aloe vera will reduce inflammation during the therapies.

An amino acid supplement of N-acetyl Cysteine containing glutamine (which stimulates the liver to produce glutathione, a natural compound that repairs damaged cells) and L-Cysteine (which is particularly important in DNA repair) may help you keep your healthy cells stable. Or you can eat lots of raw carrots, asparagus, avocado, cruciferous vegetables – broccoli, Brussel sprouts, cabbage etc – which are especially strong in glutathione; and kelp, eggs and garlic for L-Cysteine. And go out in the sunshine for your vitamin D. Remember magnesium rich foods, or supplements, soya lecithin, bold tea, dandelion and milk thistle will help de-fat and strengthen your liver during this time. And later you can rebuild your immune system with supplements like echinacea, cat's claw, total vitamin E, chlorella. And MGN-3 (Biobran) on top of the astragalus you are already taking.

There's so much more to supplements than the vast majority of doctors and the media even realise.

Key vitamins in the fight against cancer

More detailed information with references can be found at www.canceractive.com under nutritionals.

VITAMIN A

Information: Cannot be synthesised in the body. Must be ingested directly, or can be made in the body from its precursor beta-carotene. Fat soluble. Too much is highly toxic to the liver, so it is best to supplement with only a little natural vitamin A, and top up with beta-carotene allowing the body to make more if it needs it.
Sources: Oily fish is the best source. Cod liver oil supplements.
Daily anti-cancer 'dose': Female 700 micrograms; male 900 micrograms
Known benefits: Many studies show its cancer-fighting abilities. For example, it protects in breast cancer (Iowa study) and can cause remission in leukaemia (Sloan-Kettering).

BETA-CAROTENE

Information: Carotenoids and, within this group of natural compounds, beta-carotene are readily available in foods, but water soluble. So if supplements are taken, they should be with food and spread out across the day. Importantly natural beta-carotene comes in two forms (all trans, and 9-cis) – synthetic supplements tend to have just the former which may account for the poor reviews the supplement receives occasionally.
Sources: Carotenoids are typically orange/red in colour (see also lycopene). The orange pigment in carrots, peppers, apricots and pumpkins. Tomatoes, kale, cherries, sweet potato, chicory and chlorella also have good levels.

Daily anti-cancer 'dose': Normal levels are 6 mgs – but anti-cancer dosage can go to 60 mgs per day. Smokers should not take synthetic beta-carotene; there are two studies suggesting it increases risk.

Known benefits: Several prevention studies show a reduction in cancer risk by 40 per cent, using beta-carotene supplementation. Studies with colon cancer show an immune boosting effect; it increases NK cells and cancer cell inhibition.

B VITAMINS

Information: Wide range of benefits from this range of vitamins, some of which have quite individual characteristics
Sources: Primarily whole grains, but also 'greens' and nuts

Most notable components in the fight against cancer are:

FOLIC ACID

Information: Folate levels have declined by as much as 16 per cent on average in just the last 5 years according to research in MMWR. But it is essential for making perfect copies of our genetic code when cells divide or send out messages.
Source: Leafy vegetables, avocado, pulses, carrots, melon, apricots, whole grains. Its release from foods is controlled by beneficial bacteria in the colon. It is destroyed by oestrogen and oestrogen mimics.
Daily anti-cancer 'dose': 400 mgs
Known benefits: Essential for accurate copying of cellular genetic code and helps in the development of key messengers, enzymes and proteins. (It even has an anti-ageing role in the brain and also a role in heart disease.) A lack of it is noted in some cancers especially colorectal cancers.

VITAMIN B-12

Information: Essential vitamin – a lack of which is known in breast cancer, colon cancer and stomach cancers. Vegetarians also show deficiencies. A deficiency is linked with a deficiency of folic acid.
Sources: Liver, kidney, lean meat, oysters, seafood, chlorella,

although beneficial bacteria are crucially involved in its release from foods.

Daily anti-cancer 'dose': Take Chlorella, if you don't want to eat meat.

Known benefits: Involved in over 300 chemical reactions in the body, its other name is cyano-cobalmine because of its constituent molecules.

VITAMIN B-17

Information: Cannot be prescribed in the UK. Like B-12 the molecule can be broken by certain enzymes to release cyanide. These enzymes do not exist in healthy cells but only in the power systems of cancer cells. Although B-17 is much derided, pharmaceutical companies are currently working on drugs to do exactly the same job!

Sources: Apricot Kernels, pips of apples, certain nuts like cashews, pecans, macadamia and almonds, gooseberries, blackberries and other berries, barley, millet and brown rice, water cress, bamboo shoots, sweet potato, papaya.

Daily anti-cancer 'dose': Prevention experts say 6 apricot kernels a day. For people with cancer: Never take more than 6 in 90 minutes; never more than 35 in a day; and ensure you have a reasonably healthy liver..

Known benefits: Some people claim that B-17 can selectively target and kill cancer cells. There are 5 studies, 3 with animals and 2 with humans that lend some support to this view.

BIOTIN

Information: Seems to play a 'helper' role with other immune system boosters. Deficiency where beneficial bacteria activity is impaired in intestine.

Sources: Nuts, whole grains, brown rice. Beneficial Bacteria are essential for the release of biotin – it is often erroneously claimed that they 'make it'.

Daily anti-cancer 'dose': In B complex or 0.3 mgs supplement

Known benefits: Actual anti-cancer action uncertain, but seems to work as a co-factor to vitamins A, C B2, B6 and niacin. Does have a boosting effect on the immune system.

VITAMIN C

Information: Readily available; always better to eat the natural fruits and vegetables as it is in such plentiful supply and comes with co-factors, like enzymes and bioflavenoids, that help its action. It is water soluble so a little should be ingested at various times throughout the day. You won't store excess.

Sources: Best are red peppers, broccoli, papaya, berries, cauliflowers, citrus fruits, potatoes and tomatoes

Daily anti-cancer 'dose': 2gms – but up to 10 gms if you have cancer.

Known benefits: Vitamin C boosts the immune system, protects cells and cell walls from attack and, in large doses of 20-50 grams (mega-doses), helps oxygenate cancer cells by increasing glutathione levels (since cancer cells can't use oxygen, this kills them). It can also neutralise the toxins from parasites

VITAMIN D

Information: Essential vitamin to have in your prevention and treatment repertoire, although it acts more like a hormone. Great amounts of new research from the USA, especially Harvard. Cancer cells have large numbers of vitamin D receptors and the vitamin appears to kill cancer cells. Drug companies are now trying to concentrate the vitamin and patent it; for example the drug Asentar is in Stage III clinical trials – it is said to have enormous potential.

Sources: Made by the action of sunlight on the cholesterol layers below your skin. No other source comes even near this. A little is found in oily fish, and far less still in dairy.

Daily anti-cancer 'dose': Scaremongering about the negative effects of sunshine, coupled with office jobs, indoor lifestyles and gloomy weather seem to be causing a crisis. Research shows deficiencies now appearing in urban populations. Supplement with vitamin D3 which your liver will convert to the active ingredient. RDA is currently 5-6 micrograms or less than 1000 IU's but research now shows levels of 20-30 times this are perfectly safe – you will get 40,000 IU's from a day on the beach. Two megastudies from Moores Cancer Centre in San Diego have shown huge potential cancer reductions. One concludes spending 15-20 minutes and taking 2000 IU's per day would result in a 50 per cent reduction in breast cancer, while the other concludes colorectal cancers would be reduced by two-thirds if people took enough sunshine or supplements. Black people living in poor sun environments should definitely supplement.

Known benefits: Harvard say it is protective for more than 15 cancers from breast, to prostate, to colon and pancreatic cancer. Their professor (Hollick) says 25 per cent less women would die from breast cancer if they took adequate amounts. In another study which followed 1.1 million men and women for 30 years, those with higher blood levels of vitamin D had significantly less deaths from cancer. The sun belt in the USA has long been associated with lower cancer rates. It seems the sun, supported by plenty of green vegetables, really is a strong factor. It prevents – and it seems to help you beat cancer too. Research from Kings College says sunshine actually keeps you younger inside as well! Known to improve success in radiotherapy.

VITAMIN E

Information: Recent research is throwing official recommendations to the wind. There are 8 forms of vitamin E: 4 forms of tocopherols, and 4 of tocotrienols. (alpha, beta, gamma, and delta of each). The EU only officially permits the sale of synthetic alpha tocopherol, a form that may increase risk of death, reduce longevity and even block the action of beneficial tocotrienols!!

Sources: Give up crisps and bag snacks and put out bowls of seeds and nuts instead. Sunflower, pumpkin, sesame and linseeds, plus almonds and other nuts. Also found in whole grains, spinach, cabbage, lettuce, eggs.

Daily anti-cancer 'dose': Levels of this vitamin have been declining in natural foods. To get an all round benefit you should think 'total' – a totally natural vitamin E, with all the 8 forms in total. 400 IU's per day

Known benefits: Over 800 studies suggest benefit from this vitamin. It stops fats damaging the immune system by turning 'rancid'; low levels are linked to many cancers and it is a proven immune booster. A review of 12 studies in 2005 alone showed the importance of tocotrienols in beating breast cancer. Recent Japanese research shows that two forms of natural tocotrienols (alpha and delta) directly inhibit a cancer promoting enzyme (DNA polymerase), can disrupt the formation of blood vessels by tumours, and can reduce metastasis.

GLUTATHIONE

Information: A very powerful antioxidant that is produced in all cells in the body – an important part of the power production, it keeps the cell's oxygen levels up.

Sources: Widely available in fruits and vegetables; top providers are avocado, asparagus, watermelon, grapefruit, strawberries, raw tomatoes, oranges and lightly boiled or steamed cabbage, Brussel sprouts, cauliflower and broccoli.

Daily anti-cancer 'dose': Little need for supplements if you eat the above foods.

Known benefits: Older people with the highest levels of glutathione in their bloodstream, overcome illness quickest. This highlights the science behind why eating real foods is good and junk food is no good for you. It neutralises free radicals and harmful fats.

VITAMIN K

Information: Used traditionally to aid blood clotting, the RDA level set is miniscule and only three groups of researchers study it in the world. That may change.

Sources: Green leafy vegetables, broccoli. But the vitamin K cannot be released without the involvement of beneficial bacteria.

Daily anti-cancer 'dose': The RDA was set at 50 micrograms to aid blood clotting. No official recommendations on dosage – but levels of up to 500 times have been shown to be safe. Take vitamin K2 supplements or sort out your beneficial bacteria and diet. Or both!

Known benefits: First researchers in Washington and Tokyo showed that it could stop some liver cancers completely. Then a benefit was shown with leukaemia and pancreatic cancers. This is hardly surprising; 200 years ago we ate a lot of greens and we had healthy intestinal flora.

LYCOPENE

Information: An antioxidant and carotenoid, but not commonly mentioned. It binds to, and breaks up certain fats in the blood stream and tissues.

Sources: Tomatoes, tomatoes and especially cooked tomatoes which release the vitamin more readily

Daily anti-cancer 'dose': 10-15 mgs.

Known benefits: Harvard Medical School showed that eating ten helpings of tomatoes per week could reduce prostate cancer risk by 40 per cent. And if you had the cancer already, it could reduce the symptoms by 40 per cent as well. It is known to displace certain heavy metals bound in fatty tissue.

Key minerals in the fight against cancer

CALCIUM

Information: It helps regulate the power producing activities in the power stations of healthy cells; and low calcium causes a hormone calcitriol to be produced, which increases fat stores in the body. However, Gerson make the argument that calcium is in the same column of the periodic table as sodium and so will have similar effects; and they believe that too much calcium can increase cancer risk. Some cancer experts also believe this too. Calcium may cause problems directly, or excess calcium can reduce magnesium and vitamin D levels both of which protect.

Sources: Increasingly depleted in our soils calcium is in a wide range of green vegetables, grains and nuts. It is easily absorbed,

Daily anti-cancer 'dose': The issue with calcium is not intake – a helping of spinach or cabbage is enough for a day. The issue is storage and depletion. Calcium is easily absorbed, stored and re-usable as long as vitamin D and magnesium are present. Smoking, oestrogen and alcohol deplete the stores. Coral calcium and other similar organic supplements are excellent providers. A maximum intake of 1 gram per day is plenty.

Known benefits: Several studies have shown that low blood calcium levels are linked to breast and colon cancers. However, Rudolf Keller and Dr Max Gerson believe that calcium stimulated tumour growth. The Karolinska Institute has warned on dairy consumption and the Fox Chase Cancer Centre in Philadelphia has warned on its high calcium levels (May 2005). Men with the highest intake of dairy calcium are 2.2 times more likely to develop prostate cancer.

MAGNESIUM

Information: Essential mineral for the transportation of other minerals into and out of the cell. 40 per cent of adults are deficient in it.
Sources: Pulses, whole grains, 'greens', apples, pears, jacket potato, nuts.
Daily anti-cancer dose: Just eat the fresh food listed. Magnesium is available in organic supplement form.
Known benefits: Without enough magnesium, the calcium and potassium transport system into your tissues cannot function correctly, and a build up of sodium will occur, leaving the cells acid and with lower oxygen. The Karolinska Institute has shown that the higher the intake of magnesium, the lower the risk of colorectal cancer.

POTASSIUM

Information: We really should be potassium people – and we are not. We should have an intake of potassium five times greater than our intake of sodium.
Sources: Lentils, jacket potato, broad beans and peas, whole grains, nuts bananas, fresh fish, green vegetables, brown rice, carrots, apples, pears, oranges.
Daily anti-cancer 'dose': No real need to supplement unless correcting an imbalance with sodium, in which case there are organic salts available.
Known Benefits: Ensures the power stations, or mitochondria, produce their energy in a normal cell way. Without potassium they will adopt an anaerobic method and may become cancer cells.

SELENIUM

Information: Even the studies that criticise 'antioxidants' leave selenium alone. It is deficient in European diets. One of the most important anti-cancer minerals, a deficiency has been linked directly with stomach and breast cancers.

Sources: You will hear about Brazil nuts as the best source, but you need to crack these fresh yourself. Shelf lighting with see-through bags depletes the nuts of selenium and can turn them rancid. Best sources are some types of garlic, tuna and oily fish, lobster, onions, sunflower seeds, tomatoes, wheatgerm, bran, eggs and chicken breast

Daily anti-cancer 'dose': 100-200 micrograms, (never exceed 200 micrograms) Smoking and 'bad' fats deplete its levels.

Known benefits: It works to enhance the action of vitamin E as an antioxidant. It also can displace mercury, lead and cadmium from cells, and it can even help eliminate some chemicals and oestrogen mimics from the body.

ZINC

Information: It is arguable that zinc is not itself an antioxidant but it does help others like vitamins A and C do their daily jobs. It is known to accelerate healing time.

Sources: Meat, eggs. pumpkin seeds, sunflower seeds, sesame seeds, wheatgerm, brewers' yeast, shellfish and oysters. Alcohol and vitamin B-6 can deplete it. Dairy blocks its absorption.

Daily anti-cancer 'dose': Recommended levels are 15-20 mgs (there is some indication that levels above 100 mgs can cause cancer).

Known benefits: Particularly important in the fight against prostate cancer. There is some evidence that prostate cancer is linked with heavy metals and chemical toxins. The prostate is the store of zinc in men, and zinc (like selenium) can displace these toxins – or be displaced by them. White flecks on your finger nails are a sign of deficiency. Supplementation of 15 mgs a day has been found to reduce prostate cancer risk by 40 per cent.

CHAPTER 17
HERBS IN THE FIGHT AGAINST CANCER

Surrounding Hampton Court 500 years ago were not rose gardens, but herb gardens. Herbs were just a natural part of our environmental nourishment. And eating herbs helped prevent – and treat – illness. Just as poorer Asians eat all manner of green plants nowadays so did we 500 years ago.

We used herbs not merely as 'treatments' but as protection. Stuffing the chicken with sage (an astringent) and onion (an antiviral) kept the germs away.

In the 'Handbook of Organic Food Safety and Quality', various professors and scientists studying cattle have noted that they chose to graze in certain parts of fields where different types of herbs grow. And the milk contains higher levels of natural compounds like omega 3 as a result. I can imagine the same situation for humans 500 years ago. We ate those foods that surrounded us and were in season – and herbs would have been a part of our diets. Sadly this is no longer true, and our health may be paying the price.

For example, Professor Dr. Thomas Efferth from Deutsches Krebsforschungszentrum in Heidelberg has analysed 76 medicinal plants that are believed to treat malignant tumors and other such growths. Extracts from 18 of the plants were found to significantly suppress the growth of cancer cells. He describes the results as 'way above' the results you could expect from drugs.

In Europe, Herbal Medicine is legally recognised as a legitimate healthcare system under the banner of 'Traditional Medicine'. This means that where natural herbs have traditionally defined medicinal value and/or scientific research studies on them, claims can be about their specific scientific effectiveness, and their safety.

Unfortunately, this is not the case in the USA, where they are simply dietary supplements. There, scientific research is always required and, even then, claims of medical efficacy are not allowed. In my opinion, this is nonsense as it greatly compromises the worldwide acceptance of, and belief in, herbs as healing agents. As in many things, the view of Americans dominates – and here it is palpably wrong.

Not least, herbs are less likely to feature in everyday conversations on illness if they are dubbed chemicals. And if no effects can be claimed, there is no point in prescribing them and so, they must be deemed worthless. As Europeans with 4,000 years of history in treating illnesses, we know that is simply not true.

A further, but minor, complication is that when discussing health matters with European Medical Herbalists, they rarely differentiate between what you and I might call a herb (thyme) and other active ingredients from plants (e.g. Quercitin, from apples and onions). In this chapter I will try to stick to 'Herbs'!

Hoxsey

In 1988 the Office of Technology Assessment (OTA) of the United States Congress commissioned a report on the Hoxsey Therapy. It was the first federal agency to review the therapy and did it as part of a study into alternative cancer treatments. Patricia Spain Ward PhD, a medical historian from the University of Illinois, completed a background paper for Congress; this paper details the full story. You can read a full summary on our web site – here is the shortened version!

Harry M Hoxsey (1901–1974) developed and practiced a cancer treatment. Since his death Mildred Nelson, his long-time nurse and assistant, has continued his work. In 1963 Hoxsey chose a site in Tijuana, where today stands the thriving Bio-Medical Centre, home of the therapy.

Hoxsey became a healer in the 1920s. He believed that cancer was systemic – a disease of the whole body – and developed a herbal mixture to kill it off.

His first 'therapy' was in fact an external paste, made of antimony sulphide, zinc chloride, bloodroot and other occasional ingredients like arsenic sulphide, herbs and talc. With the help of Dr Frederick Mohs, a surgeon and the Dean of Wisconsin Medical School and several of its staff, he treated surface cancers that were then surgically removed with success. Hoxsey's 'red paste' and the experiments were written up extensively in the 1940s. Dr Mohs published in 1941 in the Archives of Surgery and in 1948 in the *Journal of the American Medical Association* (*JAMA*).

However the AMA attacked and attacked, even claiming that Hoxsey and Mohs had used different pastes. One report claimed that Hoxsey's active ingredient in the 1950s was arsenic, but it turned out the AMA was using an early 1920s paste! Hoxsey had developed a caustic treatment and was an ex-mining quack. Mohs was a doctor and a surgeon, and his treatment by contrast was acceptable. In fact both men were using sanguinarine, an alkaloid in bloodroot which has potent anti-tumour effects (Young 1967).

Worse, Hoxsey had an elixir for internal cancers. And he refused to tell people, especially the AMA, what was in it although he identified alfalfa, buckthorn, red clover and prickly ash he did not name the others.

Unfortunately, Harry Hoxsey's success as a healer, the wealth it created, and his refusal to divulge the exact ingredients of his elixir made him enemies in high places.

By 1950 the FDA used the courts to demand ingredient labeling and block interstate shipments. This forced Hoxsey to reveal all, and he detailed a core set of ingredients, with variant extras depending upon the individual and their type of cancer.

The basic solution was:

Cascar (Rhamnus Purshiana) and Potassium Iodide

The additions might include any of the following:
    Poke root (Phytolaeca Americana)
    Burdock root (Arctium lappa)
    Berberis root (Berberis vulgaris)
    Buckthorn bark (Rhamnus frangula)
    Stillingia root (Stillingia sylvatica)
    Prickly ash bark (Zanthoxylum Americanum)

Both the AMA and FDA dismissed the potion as *"worthless, without any therapeutic merit in the treatment of cancer"*, and did not even analyse it.

In the *JAMA* 1954 the AMA insisted that *"Any intelligent physician could testify that all these substances were worthless."* All Hoxsey's case histories at the subsequent FDA trial were dismissed as lacking in evidence and neither the FDA nor the NCI provided any detail counter evidence or laboratory trials on cancer efficacy or otherwise. Commissioner Larrick warned Hoxsey publicly in 1956.

However scientific research now does support the ingredients. For example:

- **Pokeweed** – Triggers the immune systems, increases lymphocytes and increases levels of immunoglobulin (Farnes 1964, Downing 1968).
- **Burdock** – 'Considerable anti-tumour activity' (Szeged University 1966). 'uniquely capable of reducing mutagenicity' (Morita et al 1984).
- **Burberry** – Anti-tumour activity (Hoshi et al 1976); contains lycbetaine, an anti-tumour substance (Owen 1976).
- **Buckthorn** – Anti-leukaemia substances; anthraquinone works against tumours (Kupchan 1976).

Even the least studied herbs, stillingia and prickly ash, have anti-inflammatory or anaesthetic properties and are used in European folk remedies.

An eminent US botanist, James Duke PhD of the United States Department of Agriculture, has confirmed that all of the Hoxsey herbs have known anti-cancer properties and have long been used by Native American healers to treat cancers. Even as long ago as the 1850s; Dr J W Fell of the Middlesex Hospital was using bloodroot and zinc oxide directly onto malignant growths with great effect.

Hoxsey also had his 'converts'. The Assistant District Attorney of Dallas, Al Templeton, arrested Hoxsey almost 100 times until in 1939 his brother developed a cancer and was cured by Hoxsey. Templeton became Hoxsey's lawyer.

Esquire magazine sent journalist James Burke to Texas in 1939 to write a story 'on the quack'. He stayed six weeks, wrote 'The Quack Who Cures Cancer' and became his publicist!

In 1954 an independent team of ten US physicians made a two-day inspection of Hoxsey's clinic, then in Dallas, and concluded that he was 'successfully treating pathologically proven cases of cancer, both internal and external, without the use of surgery, radium or x-ray'.

But the fact is that still the FDA and AMA have not tested the therapy! Even in 1965 Morris Fishbein, former long term editor of *JAMA* and voice of American Medicine for 40 years referred to Hoxsey as a charlatan and talked of "ghouls and cancer quacks". Patricia Ward in her report to Congress quotes this sort of attitude as setting the "low level of discourse and the emotional rather than analytical tone." Hoxsey sued Fishbein – and won.

By 1976 the Cancer Chemotherapy National Services Center researching plants used in folklore, noted that they often had anti-cancer activity.

Hoxsey's clinics were shut down in the 1950s, when even a 1953 Federal Report to the Senate stated that the FDA, AMA and NCI had organised "a conspiracy" to suppress a fair and unbiased assessment of Hoxsey's methods (The Fitzgerald Report). At the time the Dallas clinic had 12,000 patients.

Today the Bio-Medical Center combines the flexible Hoxsey formula with diet, vitamin and mineral supplements. Liquorice and red clover, used in Essiac and prominent in tests with breast cancer at Royal Marsden, are frequent herbal additions. The clinic is outpatient only. You arrive, ideally with all your reports and tests, and they see you for a day or two. You leave with enough potions and medication to last three or more months.

Dietary advice is usually to avoid foods that conflict with the herbs; like pork, carbonated drinks, alcohol, vinegar and tomatoes. Supplements include immune stimulants, yeast tablets, vitamin C, calcium and laxatives. However the clinic does offer treatments like homeopathy and even chemotherapy.

External cancers like melanoma are frequently treated, as are cancers of the blood system. There are many case histories for all cancers from breast to colon. According to Mildred Nelson, about 80 per cent of patients seen at the clinic 'benefit substantially'.

Essiac

Another 'herbal' therapy that has run the gauntlet in the USA is Essiac, an eight ingredient herbal tea. Currently Essiac is 'unapproved for marketing' in the USA. However the Resperin Corporation, the current owners of the full formula, has a special agreement with the Canadian Health and Welfare Dept. and this allows 'emergency releases of Essiac on compassionate grounds'.

So what's the fuss all about?

The original formula was given to Nurse Rene Caisse by a hospital patient who claimed her cancer had been healed some 20 years before by an Ontario Indian medicine man.

Caisse used the blend of herbs to treat patients for a number of years, setting up her own clinic in 1935 in Braceridge, Canada. Caisse's view was that it alleviated pain, and at the same time broke down nodular masses to form a more normal tissue. (Eventually the tumour would start to soften after an earlier hardening. Patients frequently reported a discharge of large amounts of pus and fleshy material as the tumour broke down.)

Her clinic was free, and by 1938 supporters tried to win Government approval for her work, failing in parliament by three votes. Nine doctors had petitioned the Canadian federal health department as early as 1926 asking that Caisse be allowed to test her cancer remedy on a broad scale. In their signed petition they testified that the herbal treatment reduced tumour size and increased life expectancy.

Caisse's own view was that, if it doesn't actually cure cancer, it does afford significant relief. Whilst in Canada, Caisse treated her own 72 year old mother with the tea under the supervision of Dr Roscoe Graham, consultant and specialist. The tea was administered 12 times a day for 10 days, and her mother lived to 90 years of age.

By 1942, without official approval and fearing arrest, Caisse shut her clinic, although she continued to treat patients at home. In 1959 at the age of seventy she went to the Brusch Medical Centre in Massachusetts, where she treated cancer patients under the watchful eye of 18 doctors. Dr Charles Brush, who treated President Kennedy amongst other members of New England's elite, reported in 1991 that he had been taking Caisse's formula since 1984 when he himself had cancer operations.

The original herbal ingredients were:

- **Burdock root** – A well-known blood purifier which has been reported by Hungarian and Japanese scientists to decrease cell mutation and inhibit tumours. It has reasonably high selenium content.
- **Sheep Sorrel** – A traditional Indian remedy for everything from eczema to ringworm; it does have an effect in herpes, ulcers and cancer seemingly by stimulating the endocrine system.
- **Slippery Elm** – Calcium, magnesium and vitamin rich, it has a healing effect on the lungs and internal organs. It also helps reduce acidity in the body.
- **Indian Rhubarb** – Very cleansing to the liver and intestinal system. It also helps transport oxygen throughout the body and has an antibiotic and anti-yeast action and reduces inflammation. In 1980 studies showed that it also had a clear anti-tumour effect.

Whilst working with Dr Brusch between 1959 and 1978, Nurse Caisse added four other herbs to the original formula. The new formula became **Essiac,** her name spelled backwards.

The four additions are:

- **Watercress** – Strong antioxidant effects, contains bioflavonoids; it is a good source of vitamin C.
- **Blessed Thistle** – A blood purifier and immune booster
- **Red clover** – The herb of Hippocrates, the flowers are currently undergoing tests for breast cancer control.
- **Kelp** – Like chlorophyll, chlorella and spirulina, kelp is a strong provider of natural minerals especially iron and calcium in an organic and easily assimilated form. Kelp is anti-bacterial and sea vegetables, in general, help reduce acidity in the body thus improving immune function.

Nurse Caisse recommended 12 – 13 cups of the infusion per day, although there are several reports of it being administered by injection. Shortly before she died she sold the 'secret' formula to the company Resperin.

Without proper clinical trials it is impossible to come to any definitive conclusion about Essiac and a degree of mythology has clouded some of the story.

What is apparent though is that the ingredients of Essiac, if nothing else, make it an excellent all round immune system booster although some ingredients do have scientific research on their anti-cancer roles.

The role of herbs in the 'eat-to-beat-cancer' diet

In chemotherapy the chemicals act on the body, the whole body, causing harm not just to the cancer cells, but actively disrupting, interfering, interrupting, and impairing in a dynamic manner many of the body's vital processes, even with many of the so-called modern 'targeted' drugs. By contrast, the body acts on herbs and this natural process, built up over thousands of years in our inter-relationships with our surrounding environments, results in the restorative, curative and yet passive influences of herbal medicine.

The fact is that our bodies have co-evolved with the plants around us for hundreds of thousands of years, and this cannot be said of drugs.

Some orthodox medical practitioners will say, 'But we do not ignore herbs' pointing, for example, to the development of the drug Taxol from the periwinkle. But, at the moment, this is a one-off. And it is a synthetic and toxic cellular killer, using but one active ingredient of the herb. It has little to do with Herbal Medicine, for it is not the use of the whole herb by the 'animal' in its natural local environment. It reflects neither synergistic evolution nor a balance with the world around us.

Others will correctly say that no single herb can cure cancer. As we continually point out, no single anything (drug, herb, vitamin) will cure cancer and it is a fool and quack who says otherwise. The whole point of this book is to try and help people cover all the bases – across the width of the cancer process. And no single herb is going to do that – although a number of herbs may well be able to cover most of the steps, if used in combination.

Immune response

A common misconception is that merely stimulating the immune system will be enough to kick out cancer. Maybe, in a few cases it will. But, by and large, the problem with cancer is two-fold – true, the immune system is weak, BUT ....the cancer evades the immune system because of the low immune system response capacity. (In English – the bad guys can't be 'seen', no matter how many good guys you produce. The issue is to make lots of good guys AND stimulate the bad guys in such a way that they appear on the radar screens.)

So, in Herbal Medicine two therapeutic requirements are essential when treating cancer – **Immuno-modulating** herbs, and **Adaptogenic** herbs, and BOTH are required to work synergistically:

Immune system components (T-cells, B-cells, Natural Killer cells, cytokines, immunoglobulins etc) may be stimulated, for example, by the use of Shitake mushroom polysaccharides or quercitin-containing foods like onions, berries, and certain herbs like echinacea and cat's claw. The body's capacity to adapt, or respond, to the increases in the immune system also needs stimulating and this can be aided by herbs such as Korean ginseng, Pau D'Arco and astragalus. There are many others.

Attacking the cancer process

Herbal Medicines have a wide variety of potent properties and certain herbs with certain properties are known to attack different steps of the cancer process.

Here is an indication of the phenomenal strength of herbs, using just a few. There is much more information on our web site. On a personal note I found that cat's claw, astragalus, turmeric (curcumin) and echinacea can be an excellent immune system re-booting combination after treatment with radiotherapy or chemotherapy. Indeed we gave this mixture to Catherine when the chemotherapy drugs had reduced her white cells to desperately low levels, and the standard immune-stimulating drugs on offer simply wouldn't work. Her white cell levels recovered in less than two weeks.

Ten natural herbal cancer fighters

1. ASTRAGALUS

Astragalus membranaceous is a truly all round anti-cancer agent. It has been around in Chinese medicine for two thousand years. It is known as 'haung qi', or chi, because it boosted natural body energy levels. It is taken from the root of a plant needing four to seven years to mature. This herb is known to boost the immune system and specifically to treat burns, abscesses and hepatitis. In Chinese hospitals it is now used to help people recover from the negative effects of radiotherapy and chemotherapy.

FDA to approve role in cancer

Its wide usage in China as an immune system booster brought interest from Europe, Japan and America. A considerable amount of detailed German and American research has confirmed its powers and potential role in cancer therapy. The FDA is currently granting it approval as an anti-cancer agent.

An excellent immune system booster

Astragalus has phenomenal immune system modulating effects. In tests at the Hiroshima School of Medicine in Japan, it was shown to directly increase B-lymphocyte and T-lymphocyte levels, interleukin and antibody production. Astragalus contains bioflavonoids, cholines, and a polysaccharide, astragalan B, amongst other active ingredients.

Astragalan B controls bacterial infection and viruses by binding to their outer membranes and weakening their internal systems. Its use as an adjunct to fight AIDS is increasingly important. But this membrane binding ability seems to make astragalus an important adaptogenic herb too 'offering up' viruses, bacteria and even cancer cells to be seen by the immune system. And in cancer therapy, where so many cancers 'hide' from the immune system this makes astragalus a natural compound of huge potential.

Improves the effectiveness of radio- and chemotherapy

One extremely important conclusion from several US studies is that astragalus seems to help the immune system differentiate between healthy cells and rogue cells, thereby boosting the body's total 'cancer fighting system'. One effect of this is the added benefit of improving the effectiveness of radiotherapy and chemotherapy treatments.

MD Anderson Cancer Center (Texas) researchers reported that cancer patients undergoing radiotherapy had twice the survival rates if they took astragalus and this prestigious cancer centre has conducted a considerable amount of research on the herb.

It should be taken with meals at a total intake of 2,000 to 3,000 mgs per day.

2. ECHINACEA – immune booster that can kill cancer cells

Generally known as an immune system enhancer for colds, the polysaccharide, arabinogalactan, in echinacea is effective in activating macrophages, interleukin and interferon with an increase in T-cell activity. It is a very powerful immune system booster, and research shows that it can stimulate the immune system to kill microbes and directly cause cancer cell death. Indeed, separate studies show that it has had positive effects with brain tumours and more work is currently being carried out.

Should not be taken for more than 8 weeks at a time as it thins the blood.

3. CAT'S CLAW (Uno de Gato) – boosting the attack

Alkaloids are very powerful natural plant compounds and there are six oxindole alkaloids in Uno de Gato bark. This natural ingredient is found in the Peruvian rain forest and China. It is known to be anti-viral, anti-inflammatory, an antioxidant and an immune stimulator – it is known to increase various white cell levels stimulating the production of Natural Killer Cells. Four alkaloids in particular boost phagocytosis where the white cells attack, wrap up and carry

163

off the rogue cells in the body – be they microbes, viruses, antigens and even cancer cells.

Research studies have shown the herb to be very powerful in its use with AIDS and cancer therapies. Research shows an action in decreasing the size of some tumours.

It can reduce the damaging side effects from radiotherapy and chemotherapy as it seems to offer protection to healthy cells and enhances the attack on, and removal of, cancer cells.

As an anti-cancer aid it can also be combined with wild yam and aloe vera forming a very strong anti-viral, anti-bacterial immune boosting force.

It has also been shown to boost the body's natural energy levels.

You should take one gram a day on an empty stomach.

4. ALOE VERA – the double-whammy

Used by the Ancient Egyptians and Greeks for bites, burns, skin lesions and 'cancers', research has shown its potency with internal usage as well.

Aloe has two principal actions.

Firstly, it contains very active polysaccharides and one in particular, acetyl mannose, boosts cytokine levels and enhances the immune response to cancer. It is known to increase levels of T-lymphocytes, and interferon. Research has also shown that it stimulates tumour necrosis factor shutting the blood supply off to tumours and also preventing tumour formation.

Secondly, aloe vera contains six or more anti-inflammatory agents. Natural compounds such as salicylate, gammelinoleic, gibberlin, sterols and amino acids tryptophan and phenylalanine all have significant anti-inflammatory benefits.

It is also anti-viral and anti-bacterial in its action.

5. WORMWOOD

In 2007 the five malaria aid charities all agreed that the Chinese herb, *Wormwood Artemisia*, did a more effective job than the anti-malarial drugs. It is strongly anti-parasitical and anti-fungal – indeed so powerful that it need only be taken for a few days to 'clean up' your blood system. It can be used to kill parasites, yeasts and microbes while leaving beneficial bacteria unharmed.

Recent research suggests that it also has an oxidative effect on the cell, and may even play a small anti-cancer role there as oxygen is the enemy of the cancer cell.

6. BERBERINE

Found in Goldenseal root and Barberry bark, has an action against pathogens (rogue invaders, like *Helicobacter pylori*) and has been shown to be stronger and more selective than antibiotics. It improves blood supply to the spleen and produces a higher immune response. It has also been shown to inhibit tumour formation.

7. SUMA ROOT

Contains 19 different amino acids and a number of trace minerals. The high germanium content boosts oxygenation at a cellular level. Suma root contains saponins, which help regulate blood sugar, and inhibit melanoma in research. It is Immuno-stimulating and inhibits cancer cell and tumour formation. Two of its ingredients have now been patented for cancer treatment by pharmaceutical companies.

8. FEVERFEW

For centuries feverfew – which has small daisy-like flowers – has been used as a tea for treating ailments like arthritis and migraine. In 2005 researchers from Rochester University in New York showed that in higher concentrations parthenolide, the active ingredient, kills leukaemia stem cells whilst leaving healthy cells intact. When the researchers compared it to the chemotherapy drug cytarabine they found in turn that the drug showed only 'modest toxicity' to the leukaemia stem cells, but 'relatively high toxicity' to the healthy cells.

The US Government has put parthenolide onto its 'Rapid Access Programme', which is a fast track designed to take experimental drugs quickly into clinical trials. Meanwhile the scientists are saying that leukaemia patients should not take feverfew (or any other herbal supplement) without consulting a doctor first. Lead scientist Dr Craig Jordan says that, anyway, a patient would not be able to take enough of it to produce an effect.

This really sums up the whole issue with herbs. Here clearly is a herb that works: Naturally toxic to a rogue cell but, as we have lived with it for thousands of years, it doesn't harm healthy cells. Next the researchers 'pan' the current drug. Is it to be withdrawn? Then they suggest that leukaemia patients could only get enough of the herb active ingredient in a new, and as yet unmade, drug – haven't they heard of tinctures? And finally you shouldn't take a herb without consulting your doctor. Considering in the USA he knows less than nothing about nutrition (according to the US Government themselves) nor supplements, and thinks herbs have no medicinal value at all as that is the medical stance in the USA, how is he going to advise you on feverfew? So ignore the natural compound that works – while you wait for a drug that might not. Brilliant.

9. NEEM

A native of Burma, and widely found throughout India, where it is called the 'Village Pharmacy'. An immune system booster, anti-fungal, anti-viral, anti-bacterial; The National Research Council in Washington said, *'It could benefit everyone living on this planet'*.

10. CARCTOL

Is a combination of 8 herbs, each with active anti-cancer ingredients. It is used as part of a strongly body-alkalising diet and must be prescribed by a qualified medical practitioner.

HERBSHIELD

Alan Hopking, who is a very experienced Herbal Medicine Practitioner, and a member of the NIMH, has developed a herbal 'mix' called Herbshield containing over 20 active ingredients. The mixture of different herbs and natural compounds has to be prescribed by a qualified herbalist. Each natural compound delivers a different effect against the individual stages of the cancer process – from improving the immune response to actually attacking and killing cancer cells. His details can be found on the CANCERactive web site.

Sadly, the mythology continues

Of course, many oncologists will throw their arms up in horror if you tell them that you are taking herbs to boost your immune response, while they are treating you with radiotherapy or chemotherapy. But the truth is that there is an enormous amount of research on herbs *per se*, and there are a number of studies showing herbs can help in protecting healthy cells, boosting the immune system, helping cancer cells be identified, and limiting side effects during such orthodox treatments. In other words, all the evidence points to herbs helping orthodox medical approaches deliver results – and the fact that MD Anderson is prepared to say that astragalus can double survival rates is indicative of this.

Recently, there have been moves in the UK to ban herb mixtures on the grounds that, although the individual herbs may have effects that are scientifically accepted, there is little research on the effectiveness or safety of mixtures.

Experienced herbalists find these attacks laughable since people have been taking combinations of herbs for centuries and, where there are conflicts, they are already well understood and documented. It also seems rather odd that medical authorities can suddenly make pronouncements like this without having spoken to the leading experts in Herbal Medicine first to find out what research exists. Indeed qualified Herbalists would have more credibility and evidence attacking the Orthodox Medical Profession – as I said earlier, the medical profession making the attacks has properly tested only 15 per cent of their drugs in clinical trials, and increasingly prescribes cocktails of four drugs or more, when the combinations have never been near a test of any sort. And these cocktails are actually causing 28 per cent of hospital admissions in the USA – and rising. 'Let he who is without blame cast the first stone'.

Anyone wishing to learn more about herbs and what they might do for particular aspects of a diet programme should visit our website and consider contacting the National Institute of Medical Herbalists (Great Britain). The members are most usually better qualified than GP's in the field of oncology.

CHAPTER 18
HELPING HORMONES

Hormones are chemical substances that deliver messages in the body. They are so powerful that they can be effective at the level of a few parts per billion. (This is why some chemicals in everyday products are so worrying – they can act like hormones in the body, and yet Government safe limits are set in parts per million – a thousand times more concentrated!!)

Three hormones have been especially indicated in cancer prevention activities: Melatonin, Human Growth Hormone and DHEA.

All three peak in production terms in our bodies around the age of sixteen. Their volumes then decrease dramatically as we reach our fifties. Albert Einstein was being philosophical when he opinioned *"The tragedy of life is what dies inside a man when he lives."* But he could have been talking about these three essential hormones.

Melatonin

Poor sleep – a carcinogen

Melatonin is produced by your pineal gland, which sits underneath your brain, about 90 minutes after you go to sleep in a darkened room. It helps to push you into a deeper sleep.

This is a crucial hormone in the fight against cancer. Changes in blood melatonin levels are reflected in changes in the levels of two cancer stimulating hormones: IGF-1 and oestrogen, both of which rise as melatonin levels fall.

A number of studies have shown that people who have sleep deprivation, or irregular sleep patterns, have a much higher risk of cancer. For example, night shift nurses and airline hostesses have a much higher incidence of breast cancer than the norm. So much so that the International Agency for Research on Cancer (IARC), the foremost international body on the disease, is considering officially labeling night-shift work as a "probable" human carcinogen.

169

The Royal Commission on Environmental Pollution has also made a clear link between exposure to light at night and cancer. Never sleep with a light on and try to have thick dark curtains if light from outside is coming into your bedroom. They have confirmed that cancer in general has been shown to be 60 per cent more common amongst night-shift workers, and that there is even a similar risk increase among women who stay up late more than two or three times a week. Conversely, totally blind women are only half as likely to contract cancer.

Most interesting was research from the National Cancer Institute and the National Institute of Environmental Health in the United States where human breast cancer tumours were grafted on to rats. In the early hours of the morning, the rats were then given blood which had been previously taken, either from women during normal darkened-room, full sleep, or from women sleeping in artificial light conditions. The blood taken in darkness slowed the growth of the tumours by 80 per cent, whilst that taken after exposure to light accelerated it.

EMF's – the same effect

While important cancer bodies rush to dub 'night shift working' carcinogenic, officialdom still ignores the issue of Electromagnetic Fields, or EMF's for short. Although the UK Government does urge caution on living within 200 yards of power cables or child use of mobile phones, little is said about telephone masts and WiFi and other such sources. Yet if you read the Government's own review board booklet, which resulted from a study of all the research to date (some 400 studies were chosen) you would quickly conclude that EMF's deplete melatonin levels in just the same way as a lack of sleep, with an identical knock-on effect to higher IGF-1 and oestrogen levels in the body. Clusters of cancer cases around phone and other masts are increasingly observed and in South Korea the Government has ordered the dismantling of 1,500 such masts because of these concerns over 'health risks' including cancer.

Melatonin – three powerful benefits

Melatonin 'works' in a number of ways, three of which are vital to beating cancer:

- It is a hormone and stimulates the thymus gland to produce immune cells which seek and destroy rogue cells.
- It is also a know antioxidant and free radical neutraliser.
- It depresses levels of oestrogen, and IGF-1.

You can incorporate certain foods within your diet to stimulate the precursors of melatonin (I will tell you more later) but frankly the simplest thing is to supplement. Levels of 3–6 mgs are the doses usually taken, and levels of 10 mgs and above have been known to cause hallucinations.

Such supplements are easily obtained in the USA where synthetic melatonin can be purchased in most supermarkets. However in the UK and Europe the open sale of these hormone supplements is banned, although like HRT they can be prescribed. However, I doubt that your doctor fully understands the importance of melatonin, probably merely thinking that it helps you sleep better.

There is also some concern that synthetic melatonin loses its potency before most people finish the bottle. And anyway, as readers know, I am quite against synthetic supplements and especially synthetic hormones.

Better would be to try a plant melatonin – there is a very good source, called Asphalia, grown with Government grants in Wales.

Meanwhile, steer clear of EMF's and get a good night's sleep in a darkened room away from all artificial lights, power points, electric appliances, electric blankets, computers and TV's.

Human growth hormone (Hgh)

Hgh is also produced about ninety minutes after falling asleep. Its production peaks at puberty and declines to almost zero in your fifties. The good news is you can generate more by going to the gym. Hgh production can be stimulated by resistance training at almost any age when the muscles are overworked and 'tear' slightly.

Hgh helps mobilise and burn fats and stimulates the conversion of protein into lean muscle. Most importantly it also stimulates the production of the seek-and-destroy immune cells.

Even after fifty years of age, diet can also restimulate Hgh production. The amino acids argenine, tyrosine and ornithine will increase its production but in fact there is a whole set of amino acids and vitamins and minerals required for best results (argenine, tyrosine, ornithine, tryptophan and glycine work synergistically with vitamins like the B vitamins, vitamin C and minerals zinc, calcium, magnesium and potassium).

Argenine in found in nuts, brown rice, oatmeal, raisins, seeds, meats and wholemeal bread. It is interchangeable in the body with ornithine. Argenine production (from the pituitary) ceases in adults around the age of thirty. Trauma will also stop its production.

It is very interesting to note that calorie restriction limits insulin production and also stimulates Hgh production, having the double benefit of controlling negative hormones whilst aiding the levels of this significant cancer fighter.

DHEA (dehydroepiandrosterone)

This is a natural hormone produced by the adrenal glands. Again its production declines with age. It is protective against free radicals and some people use DHEA supplements although results are very mixed and some increased cancer risks have been noted. It seems to be weakened by oestrogen and stimulated by progesterone. Wild yam acts as a precursor and natural stimulator of DHEA (as for progesterone), and has also been shown to be an excellent booster of the immune system.

Based on the very mixed results from the research I have read, I'm not too sure that people should be supplementing with this hormone at all. However it has its fans in the USA.

Thyroxin – poorly understood

Finally, I want to mention **thyroxin**, the hormone of the thyroid gland. Again, it's one of the hormones that declines with age. Importantly, it controls your metabolism. High thyroxin levels increase your metabolism. With low levels you put on weight and become easily tired and listless.

Thyroxin came to my attention because I received Personal Prescription application forms from three very different women, of different backgrounds, age and physical appearance. All had breast cancer and all were taking synthetic thyroxin prescribed by their Doctor because of poor thyroid function.

Co-incidentally, I received research from the USA which said that women with poor thyroid function had <u>less</u> cancer risk. So I did my homework. Sure enough, if you have an impaired thyroid, and therefore lowered natural thyroxin production, the research indicates you develop less cancer. It's not surprising really, is it? With high thyroxin you'd expect higher metabolic rates and more free radicals, waste products and toxins.

Thyroxin shares similar pathways with oestrogen. What surprised me was that the fat short patient was taking the same levels of daily thyroxin supplement as the thin short one and the thin tall one. Exactly the same daily dose?! Can this be right? And then I found research in America dating back over 30 years which warned that people should be careful taking synthetic doses of thyroxin as it increased metabolism and increased cancer rates. I published a paper on my monthly e-newsletter. It brought protests from two doctors. Apparently different levels of thyroxin are supposedly prescribed depending upon age, weight, sex and even weather conditions, they claimed. All I could reply was that in the case of my three ladies that simply was not true.

A further complication, quoted in the American research, was that too few doctors investigate why someone has low thyroxin production. One possible explanation is a low intake of iodine. Levels of iodine are important to thyroxin production and some diets are deficient in iodine.

If that was the underlying but undiagnosed cause, and you are encouraged to take a standard dose of synthetic thyroxin supplement, but then have an iodine rich dinner (oysters, shellfish), you can easily end up with too much thyroxin in your blood stream and a heightened metabolism. And you wouldn't want that at all. It would increase your risk of cancer.

If you have a problem with your thyroid, please make your first port of call a nutritionist or naturopath or other diet expert.

Summary

I am not a fan of synthetic supplements, especially synthetic hormone supplements. I've read the research on HRT!

So, I suggest that you would be wise to steer clear of EMF's as much as possible and, if over 50 years of age, to supplement with asphalia. And you should always sleep in complete darkness (and so should your children).

A regular visit to the gym would do no harm where you might try lifting a few weights under supervision.

I think an annual visit to a specialist nutritionist would be no bad thing either. You service your car once per year – why not yourself?

SECTION 2

RE-BUILDING A LIFE

"Life is something that happens when you can't get to sleep."
(Fran Lebowitz)

And there is a fair summation of the problem at large. Too many people seem to think of life as passive – it's something that happens. Getting cancer is just bad luck.

This attitude, by and large, is rubbish.

You get out of life what you put in, and nowhere is this more true than with your health. Of course, genetics plays some part; and even your wealth, or lack of it. But by now you will have seen that even the poorest people can be happy, healthy and avoid cancer. The problem is that life in the West is 'broken', with toxicity everywhere, stresses, sedentary jobs and nutritionally deficient, non-nourishing foods.

And so you have to build your own micro-climate; your own little protective cocoon. You need to maximise your immune system, cut out the dangers and nourish your body – we've already seen what the issues are.

Now it's time to start to prepare some plans.

CHAPTER 19
EAT-TO-BEAT OESTROGEN?

Fuelling the fire of cancer

A large number of cancers, both male and female, are hormonally responsive and the prime culprit is often oestrogen. Oestrogen fuels the fire of cancer and it seems to act in a number of ways.

Earlier in the book we saw two theories of cancer formation:

* Where oestrogen can cause stem cells to stay in their rapidly dividing trophoblast state.
* Where an aggressive member of the oestrogen family, oestradiol, can sit on cellular membrane receptor sites directing havoc inside the cell – increasing cellular sodium levels, lowering oxygen levels, creating an acid environment and reducing the cells energy and repair systems.

Oestrogen may act in many other ways to propagate human cancers. For example:

* Oestrogen is known to help cancer messages bind to receptor sites on cells, thus spreading the cancer. Indeed, it has been known to cause and spread cancers since the mid 1990's (NCI). When oestrogen is added to cancer cells *in-vitro*, those cells proliferate (Dr Anna Soto, Tufts Cancer Center).
* In excess, it reduces zinc levels in the body (the prostate, for example, is a store of zinc and low zinc levels are associated with increased risk of cancer).
* It destroys folate and biotin, both vitamins essential in DNA replication and the immune system.
* It weakens the insulin control of blood glucose – the food of the cancer cell.

Excess oestrogen is linked to cancers in both males and females from melanomas to ovarian, from prostate to colon.

Oestrogen excess has been linked to other problems in the body and resultant diseases. For example, water retention, osteoporosis, fatigue, memory loss, increases blood clotting and histamine levels, along with allergies, depression, dry skin and even to diseases like Alzheimer's!

What is oestrogen?

Oestrogen is a hormone and has a number of important roles in the body, primarily being concerned with the reproductive cycle. Levels of oestrogen increase during the first two weeks of the female 'cycle', decreasing in the second two weeks as the balancing hormone, progesterone, increases its levels.

In men, oestrogen levels increase, as testosterone levels decline, over the age of 55 or so.

Oestrogen is actually not a single 'item' – it is a family of hormones all capable of binding to receptor sites on cell membranes – be they healthy or unhealthy cells, stem cells or cancer cells. The aggressive sister is normally referred to as 'oestradiol'. Then there is a weaker sister called oestrone, which is about 40 times less aggressive when it alights on the cellular receptor sites. Far weaker still are the plant 'oestrogens', called phytoestrogens. In fact experts now believe that the high levels of phytoestrogens in the blood streams of South East Asian people actually protect the individuals by binding to the receptor sites, and blocking the ability of oestradiol to take up the same position. This blocking action is also the theory behind Tamoxifen, the breast cancer drug.

The fact is that the 'oestrogen pool' is far larger in our bodies than ever before and it's killing us. (We have a book specifically on the subject detailing the best ways of cutting your oestrogen levels – *'Oestrogen: The Killer in Our Midst'*.) Cancer Research UK recently estimated that blood oestrogen levels were growing by seven per cent per year in women! And breast cancer is growing by two to three per cent.

Which takes us to a fourth group of oestrogens, that the drug sponsored charities seem to deny exists: Dr Soto also showed that there is a large number of chemicals, found in everyday toiletries, cosmetics, perfumes and household cleaners, disinfectants, plastic bottles and packaging, but also in fertilisers and pesticides that once inside our bodies can mimic the action of oestrogen. These are often termed oestrogen mimics or xeno-oestrogens. She has also proven, worryingly, that their effects can even be cumulative.

Oestrogen levels are rising in our bodies, whether from our own natural hormones, ingested animal versions, synthetic copies like HRT, or from these chemicals that 'mimic' its action.

Each week people ring our magazine **icon** to ask about breast cancers, prostate cancers, colon cancers, melanoma and even rare cancers like Hurtle's cells, all of which have been linked with high oestrogen levels. Many more cancers are linked to this same hormone, even some lung and brain cancers.

Although it is relatively easy for a woman to understand that oestrogen might be involved in her cancer, men find it hard to believe that this 'female' hormone could have anything to do with theirs. However it is clearly implicated in, for example, both prostate and testicular cancers.

Let us start with the most obvious link:

Oestrogen and breast cancers

The Bush people of the Kalahari Desert in Africa have a diet largely from vegetable sources with the odd, lean and usually small animal as a treat. Of course, they also have no stress, pollution and electro-magnetic radiation to worry about. Seven per cent of their population is over 65 years of age. They have worn but not bad teeth, whilst in some parts of Europe a third of the population has no teeth at all. They eat little or no animal fat and never dairy from cows. And they have no breast cancer.

Breastfeeding is the norm and continues until the child is four to five years old. In the West some mothers do not breastfeed their children at all, whilst many rarely exceed six months.

In August 2002 Cancer Research UK published the definitive study on breastfeeding and breast cancer.

It concluded that **the more time a women spends breastfeeding in her life, the less her own risk of breast cancer.**

Scientists have also shown that **the fewer menstrual cycles a woman goes through in her life, the lower her chance of breast cancer.**

Scientists have long been concerned in the West about the lengthening years of fertility in women, a fact that has its roots in our diets. One hundred and fifty or more years ago, a woman was likely to have been fertile from the age of 16 to her late thirties. Without contraception she may have had four children, and these she would have breastfed for nine months or more. The current New York female may have menstrual cycles lasting from her twelfth to her fiftieth birthday, and have two or less children en route. This increases her total number of periods from around 200 to as many as 440. And that's a lot more monthly oestrogen surges and resultant hormone fluctuation. Scientists believe this is also reflected in, for example, increasing incidence of endometriosis and polycystic ovary syndrome.

The Collaborative Group on Hormonal Factors in Breast Cancer, supported by Cancer Research UK, published findings in the *Lancet* in late July 2002 on 'Breast Cancer and Breastfeeding'.

Having reviewed over 50,000 women with breast cancer and 97,000 without, in 47 studies across 30 countries they concluded that the relative risk of breast cancer decreased by 7 per cent for each birth, plus 4.3 per cent for every 12 months of breastfeeding.

These figures seem to apply whether one is studying a developed, or a developing country.

In the report the main reason given for these findings confirmed that, 'the more periods a woman has, the greater her overall oestrogen production during her lifetime. Oestrogen is known to have a negative effect on the breast tissue causing it to become dense. And dense breast tissue is risky breast tissue.'

The report finished by stating that there were about 470,000 women in developed countries with breast cancer, and if women had 2.5 children on average and breastfed each for 12 months longer than they currently do, about 11 per cent (50,000) breast cancers would be prevented annually (Valerie Beal, Cancer Research UK, Epidemiology Unit).

Worse, **modern women add to their levels of oestrogen by taking the pill or HRT**. Again Cancer Research UK published data that showed women who take the pill increase their chances of breast cancer by 26 per cent. If they take it into their thirties this extra risk rises to 58 per cent. For the 10 per cent of women who take it into their 40s, the figure increases to 144 per cent.

It is worth noting that the original FDA approval for the pill was granted following a single trial on 132 Puerto Rican women, despite five of them dying during the trial (*Science* 259, 1993 Marshall). This resulted in a newer, safer pill in the 70s with a lower dose of oestrogen. However, to this day, there is no single long-term trial showing the pill to be safe.

HRT is a similar though weaker oestrogen-based pill. The late doctor John Lee, who spent more than twenty years looking into oestrogen and its effects on the body, was clear that 'too much oestrogen relative to natural progesterone levels' is the essence of the problems facing women at menopause. He showed that oestrogen at menopause merely fell from 100 per cent to around 65 – 70 per cent, or just enough to switch off egg production. Whereas the real 'faller' was natural progesterone which fell from 100 per cent to less than 3 per cent. Arguably with the increases in blood oestrogen being shown by Cancer Research UK, the last thing a post menopausal woman needs is more oestrogen. Yet women are routinely told they need more oestrogen, and HRT is prescribed to 'alleviate menopausal symptoms'!

In 2002, a seven-year HRT trial, part of the US Women's Health Initiative study, was stopped when the dangers started to emerge. The part of the trial involving a mixed synthetic oestrogen and progesten pill had resulted in a doubling of breast cancer risk.

The part of the trial using an oestrogen-only pill was allowed to continue, but 2.2 million women in the UK may have read that their risk of breast cancer rises by at least 27 per cent solely by taking oestrogen-based HRT.

Other cancers that also might develop were not recorded in this report but The Boston Nurses Study report in 1995 warned of the same risk – 27 per cent increase for breast cancer – but went on to conclude that there was significant risk of other cancers like ovarian too, depending upon length of usage.

The UK Million Women study in 2003 confirmed the increased breast cancer risks, and the German Health minister even went on to say that HRT was 'the new thalidomide'!

Part of the problem is not just the added oestrogen to the body, but the use of synthetic hormone. All synthetic products will have side effects to some degree, even vitamin pills. And of particular concern is synthetic progestin, often confused by the Medical Profession with natural progesterone. Synthetic Progesten has a number of research studies pointing the finger of danger in its direction, whereas natural progesterone actually reduces cancer risks.

If HRT were a herbal supplement, it would have been banned within a week. Interestingly, even the pharmaceutical companies list over 100 potential problems associated with HRT. The one thing they don't tell you is that oestrogen supplementation can be addictive. The *British Medical Bulletin* (1992: 48) talks about problems for women wishing to stop HRT after long-term treatment!

Oestrogen and male cancers

Several studies have linked **Testicular cancer** to xeno-estrogens. For example, in December 2002, Swedish researchers showed that three quarters of perfumed toiletry products tested contained oestrogen mimics and once in the body, levels of DEHP increased. Perfumes, perfumed body sprays, hairsprays and hair products were the main culprits. Research with pregnant women showed that DEHP affected at least 11 per cent of the male offspring, causing reproductive health problems including undescended testicles, smaller organ size and even to increased levels of testicular cancer.

In **Prostate cancer** patients are routinely told that the cause is 'high testosterone'. This is tosh. If high testosterone caused prostate cancer, the world would be full of 16 year old male patients.

As men age their testosterone level declines but their oestrogen level increases.

Oestradiol can cause enlargement of the prostate gland – anti-oestrogens, for example, Finistride and ICI, can reduce it. Oestradiol can then convert nice safe testosterone to nasty aggressive DHT, which actually sets off the cancer chain reaction

(Thompson, Texas Cancer Center). Research from Singapore National Cancer Centre, the Concord Cancer Institute, Sydney and the Monash Cancer Centre in Australia has confirmed that this 'oestrogen plus testosterone' combination is the usual methodology.

Of course, flooding your body with oestrogen via pills and injections may temporarily stop testosterone production altogether, and thus one of the two precursors of DHT will be removed. But how long is it before the body fights back? The healthy body is in a state of homeostasis – its hormones are balanced. Throw this out, cut one to nothing, and your body will try to correct by doing everything in its power to replace the missing testosterone. Taking oestrogen supplements is no long-term solution. And sadly doctors and patients alike know this now. (See Chapter 10, Professor Ben Pfeifer)

Oestrogen and other cancers

Birmingham University has shown that colorectal cancer is associated with localised oestrogen. Cervical cancers, ovarian cancers and endometrial/womb cancers are too. (In fact, there is a link between Tamoxifen and increased risk of womb cancer). Stomach cancer has been shown to be linked to oestrogenic activity on stem cells by British Columbia University as has brain cancer and gliomas (MD Anderson).

So how could diet help?

Many women with oestrogen driven cancer are given drugs like Arimidex and other Aromatase Inhibitors to cut their hormone levels and prevent their cancer growing or returning. If you could do it by diet, wouldn't that be smarter?

- Eating high fat and protein diets increases oestrogen levels.
- Eating excess calories and high sugar content increase oestrogen levels.
- Being overweight increases oestrogen levels
- Localised electrical fields (EMF's) can increase oestrogen levels
- Poor sleeping patterns can increase oestrogen levels

BUT

- Eating certain foods can reduce aggressive oestrogen levels coverting it to less aggressive forms
- Eating certain foods can block the action of some oestrogens even changing the receptor sites
- Having a healthy intestinal 'bacterial' flora can eliminate oestrogens, even synthetic ones, with the help of certain fibrous foods
- Sleeping better and eating natural compounds can reduce oestrogen levels

The diet factor

Our diets and the way we live and eat cause excesses of oestrogen. For example:

1. *High calories, high oestrogen*

A high fat, high sugar and high refined carbohydrate diet provides high calories, and the sugars will flood the blood stream. Worse, we no longer graze, we eat one or two big meals a day, concentrating the period of the sugar rush. High sugar rushes cause high insulin levels, as the body has to cope with high blood sugar levels and stop it getting to the brain and causing damage. Insulin surges completely throw out the balance between all the hormones in the body and one in particular also surges – oestrogen. High sugar levels are also linked to cancer promotion. High fat intake also heightens steroid levels, which increase oestrogen levels too.

- A five to ten per cent reduction in daily calorie intake reduces oestrogen levels by 20 per cent.
- Practice portion control.
- Graze – eat six small meals per day.
- Eat slowly.
- Eat whole foods – not refined.

2. *Being overweight*

Right at the start of the book I warned that being more than 7 kilograms overweight can seriously reduce your life expectancy, being linked to increased risk of heart disease and cancer.

One reason for this is that fat is an excellent solvent and will dissolve and store, all manner of toxins and hormones (like oestrogen) your body would rather have excreted. Another reason is that your own fat stores are the raw materials for oestrogen production.

North Carolina University have research that shows reducing your weight does reduce your risk of cancer, and increases your survival time if you have it already. So what are you waiting for?

3. *Phytoestrogens*

Human oestrogen control

In 1900 we derived 30 per cent of our protein in England from pulses – 100 years on it is just 2 per cent.

And pulses protected us, along with our large consumption of fruit and vegetables. They produced large amounts of phyto-estrogens in our blood streams. These substances are much weaker than human oestrogens, competed with it and helped control its levels and effects.

For example, research shows in women with high genistein levels (a phytoestrogen), menstrual cycles are elongated, more regular and reduced in number. This is a good thing. Women in the Far East have blood genistein levels up to one thousand times those of New York women. But we could have these protective levels too. Just remember the foods that have protected us in the UK for centuries: Pulses, broad beans, peas, lentils, chickpeas, plus vegetables like parsnips, turnips, carrots, red peppers, toma-toes and 'greens' like cabbage, Brussel sprouts and broccoli, and herbs. All increase your phytoestrogen levels.

You can think of phytoestrogens as much, much weaker cousins of oestradiol, and decide which one you would rather have sitting on your cellular oestrogen receptor sites. Or like some experts you can think of phytoestrogens as 'anti-oestro-gens'. Professor Trevor Powles, former head of the breast cancer unit at the Royal Marsden Hospital and a patron of CANCER-active calls them anti-oestrogens too and is quite clear on their benefits. At the Royal Marsden they are researching the benefits of red clover (high in genistein) with cancer patients. Red clover, the herb of Hippocrates, gives even richer levels of certain phytoestrogens and Professor Powles is confident that they will find a level of usage that is successful with cancers.

Another anti-oestrogenic constituent of vegetables, lignan, is found in high concentrations in the urine of Eastern populations who eat high vegetable diets, especially unrefined grains, seeds, pulses and legumes. The same populations excrete high levels of isoflavenoids (particularly genistein and daidzein). And there is a strong correlation between this and decreased breast cancer rates.

A typical current Western diet of high calories, high saturated fat and high protein by contrast has a double negative: Not only does it elevate the sex hormone oestrogen levels; it decreases the 'Sex Hormone Binding Globulin', which would have helped remove them from the body. A diet high in isoflavenoids, flavenoids, lignans and other such phytoestrogens has three research-proven benefits:

- It redresses this imbalance.
- It been clearly shown to block receptor sites on the cell for the mammalian sex hormone oestradiol.
- It can even reduce the growth-inducing protein tyrosine kinase in the cells.

Downgrading dangerous oestradiol

Another important benefit of natural compounds in foods is that they can also **'downgrade'** aggressive oestradiol to its safer sisters:

- **Resveratrol** from grapes, **quercitin** from onions, **prunetin** from plums and cherries and **indole-3-carbinol,** from broccoli and cabbages, are all natural substances shown in research to alter the way oestrogen is metabolised in the body, changing it (downgrading it) from the form, oestradiol, that promotes cancer cell formation to its much safer-sister product, oestrone.
- Flaxseeds, when used as a concentrate, have been shown in research to stop the growth of breast cancer, even reducing the size of breast tumours in rats by 50 per cent.

186

All of these will be covered in more detail in Chapter 24. I will give just one example of the power of natural compounds here.

Indole-3-carbinol (I3C) is emerging as a very important natural compound in the 'treatment' of oestrogen driven cancers. It has been dubbed 'The Safer, Natural Tamoxifen'. According to scientists at Leicester University, I3C also seems to actually alter some of the receptor sites preventing the action of oestradiol. It was shown by UCLA to inhibit the growth of oestrogen-positive breast cancer cells by 90 per cent (Tamoxifen scores 60) and also to detoxify the by-products of oestradiol breakdown (Tamoxifen has no action).

Moreover, the Strang Cancer Research Institute has shown it can even breakdown the by-products produced from chemical oestrogens, mimics or xenoestrogens.

I3C affects enzymes involved in the cancer process, and has been shown to stop the growth of cancer cells and also kill them. Not surprisingly, pharmaceutical companies are trying to patent synthetic versions of this natural compound.

Soya is nowadays perhaps one of the most talked about contributors of phytoestrogens in the West, but I would rather you focussed on the 500 other natural vegetables and fruits that have protected us in the Western World for the last 20,000 years – foods we just don't eat in the volumes we did.

A lot of confusion exists when it comes to soya. Most usually this confusion is caused by a squabble between advocates and adversaries of dairy and soya, frankly, some of whom are paid by the respective industries. Be clear – in this chapter I'm not talking about soya – I'm talking about foods in general that provide phytoestrogens.

Readers will undoubtedly want to know the truth about soya – my view is that we have plenty of European phytoestrogen-rich foods to eat without becoming hung up on one from the Far East. There are active ingredients that soya contains also in broad beans and peas, and so they all could be helpful. However soya is a new food to the West and I'm not at all surprised that it can cause allergies in the young, especially when already GM soya is common place.

In July 2002, Cancer Research UK published research findings on the clear benefits of soya. A study involving two new pieces of research between Cancer Research UK, The National University of Singapore and the US National Cancer Institute found that a diet rich in soya products could affect the make-up of breast tissue, potentially reducing breast cancer.

Women in the Far East who consume the most soya are 60 per cent less likely to have dense breast tissue. And dense tissue is clearly associated with an increased risk of breast cancer. The study's co-author, Dr Stephen Duffy of Cancer Research UK's Mathematics, Statistics and Epidemiology Department in London says: *"There has always been a question mark over a connection between soya and breast cancer. Some studies have suggested a link but others haven't. This research shows for the first time how the amount of soya a woman eats may have an effect on breast tissue and in turn may potentially reduce her risk of breast cancer."*

In Asian women, menopausal symptoms are almost unheard of, and they have half the levels of oestradiol and oestrone circulating in their bodies. The phytoestrogens in soya have been closely linked to lowering circulating oestradiol levels (Lee-Jane Lu) and men get less prostate and women less breast and endometrial cancers. Phytoestrogens from soya and other vegetables have been shown to be especially protective in prostate cancer (*Lancet* 1993: 342).

But please don't merely swap your large daily intake of dairy for an equivalent of soya. Soya is a new product in the Western world. If people can have wheat allergies to a product that has only been around for 10,000 years, it is no wonder we are seeing child reactions to soya, and other complications. Soya milk has been with us barely 60 years in the UK.

There is one caveat in all this – Asian women take more natural exercise. And as I said earlier, the latest research suggests regular daily exercise lowers oestrogen levels too.

4. Chemicals, pesticides and oestrogens

Many pesticides and herbicides have ingredients which, once inside our bodies, can act as oestrogen mimics. Whether we eat them directly due to their residue in our foods, or we eat the animals that ate them, hardly matters. DDT, DDE, dieldrin, lindane, methoxychlor, benzene hexachloride, kepone and more than fifty others are widely used in the world's food production and all have the ability to mimic oestrogen in the body.

The animal fat we consume from meat and dairy brings with it both oestrogens from the animals themselves plus these oestrogen mimics from the toxins in the fields. And fat makes steroids makes oestrogen.

The mimics enter the body and 'lock on' to cellular receptor sites interfering with a host of biochemical processes and making them hard to excrete. Such action has been associated with everything from brain deficiencies to reduced sperm counts, even cellular DNA interference (*Lancet* 1993) and folic acid depletion (Moscow Cancer Institute).

Dioxins are toxic chemicals so dangerous their safe levels are measured in trillionths of a gram. They activate cancer genes and suppress tumour-supressor genes.

But again, hope is at hand in the form of natural compounds from foods: For example, UCLA, Berkeley, has shown that indole-3-carbinol can affect non-oestrogen but cancer-promoting receptor sites on cells, preventing the growth of breast cancer. These sites (Ah receptors) are particular 'attacked' by chemical toxins, like dioxins. Dioxins stimulate cancer by promoting IGF-1, oestrogen and insulin levels. And I3C blocks the receptor site that dioxins attack.

Researchers at Texas University treated breast cancer cells with dioxins and I3C simultaneously and found I3C reduced the negative effects by 90 per cent. Several other studies have shown that I3C can have the effect of reducing chemically promoted breast and prostate cancers by 70 to 96 per cent.

Researchers at Tufts have shown that curcumin (turmeric) can enhance the action of phytoestrogens to inhibit aggressive human and synthetic oestrogens.

So, can you eat-to-beat chemical oestrogen mimics?

There is considerable help at hand from natural compounds. As shown above, indole-3-carbinol and curcumin and plant isoflavones can be extremely helpful, and you may remember from Chapter 15 that beneficial bacteria can break up even synthetic oestrogenic compounds.

5. *Water and oestrogen*

One of the biggest sources of unwanted oestrogen for men and women is tap water in large cities where the water is recycled.

With millions of women on the pill and HRT relieving themselves into a city's water supplies and little attention paid to filtration of the hormone, recycled tap water has become more than a little risky. Links to male genital problems have been made in several scientific studies (for example, Athlone Institute, Ireland).

We have covered water in depth in Chapter 12. To summarise the key points that affect your oestrogen levels: The best solution is to drink from glass bottled mineral water. And to use another alternative, much used in South East Asia, namely reverse osmosis filtered water to wash pans and foods, and cook with.

6. *Oestrogen in the home*

Although beyond the scope of this diet book, it is worth noting here that oestrogen mimics surround us. The average American woman has a toxin level in her bloodstream four times that of her male equivalent!

Toluene and other chemicals in perfumed soaps, perfumed this and that, and perfumes themselves are oestrogen mimics.

Cosmetics, from face creams to lipsticks, can all contain oestrogen mimics. Of course, you assume the skin prevents them getting into the blood stream – far from it. Skin is a carrier, not a barrier. The insides of your mouth, underneath your nails, your scalp and your armpits are all good absorption areas. All this makes toxins in hair dyes, nail polishes, toothpastes and deodorants easily absorbed. Worse, chemicals like sodium lauryl sulphate in soaps, bubble bath, shower gels, shampoos etc can increase the permeability of the skin by up to 40 per cent. This just allows more toxins to pass into the bloodstream.

In a German study, endometriosis was linked to chemicals called PCBs and cases of vaginal and cervical cancers have been linked to nonylphenols, which are oestrogen mimics often used in spermicides and contraceptive jellies.

Clearly men are not immune from this – they wash their faces with perfumed soap, use perfumed shaving foam and aftershave or perfumed sprays and deodorants every day.

But it doesn't end there. Your home is a toxic centre – especially if you like cleaning! Bleaches, household cleaners, nice smelling sprays, polishes add to the contamination. Volatile organic carbons can be ingested on dust particles and can come from glues holding carpet or ceiling tiles and even from petrol fumes while filling the car; or from inks in fax machines or computer circuitry if your office is not properly ventilated.

No wonder that women who stay at home have 40 per cent more toxins in their bloodstreams than their sisters who go out to work! It makes Dr Soto's finding that these oestrogen mimics can be cumulative very worrying.

It's very easy to see how we increase our 'oestrogen pool levels'. Unfortunately Governments and cancer charities aren't like the rest of us and do not condemn these products so levels of blood oestrogens will just go on rising.

Build your own clean micro-environment – men and women should ensure that they find a reputable provider of toxin-free products for their cosmetic, toiletry, cleaning and bathroom needs. In our travels we have found one company that seems to do all of this; the only company recommended in the USA by the Cancer Prevention Coalition – Neways.

7. *Oestrogen increases, and sleep*

As we observed in Chapter 18, disturbed sleep patterns are associated with increased cancer rates. Night shift workers, nurses, long-haul airline hostesses, people who sleep in artificially lit rooms – all have higher rates of cancer. And IARC are even thinking of dubbing night shift work carcinogenic'!

The fact is that poor sleep reduces melatonin levels in the body, and melatonin has a controlling influence over both IGF-1 and oestrogen levels.

Melatonin levels also decline as we age.

And melatonin levels are depleted by EMF's.

Melatonin supplements are only available on prescription in the UK. This is particularly stupid as I know of two breast cancer professors who take it but bring their own personal supplies in from the USA (which you are allowed to do). You should take no more than 3 mgs. A good alternative is the natural plant form asphalia. This is available in the UK and details are on our website.

But you can 'eat-to-increase' you melatonin as well! Eating pure dark chocolate an hour before bed will increase serotonin levels – serotonin is the precursor to melatonin. Green leaves, bananas, peanuts, dates and other protein foods like turkey and fish contain the essential amino acid tryptophan and this increases serotonin levels. Eating magnesium-rich foods and taking a supplement of B vitamins will help production too.

Remember alcohol and caffeine are poor sleep initiators.

8. *Beneficial Bacteria*

In Chapter 15 I told you about one of the biggest discoveries of this millennium: The crucial and multi-faceted role of beneficial bacteria – not just as directors of our immune systems, but in terms of helping remove toxic products from our bodies. A combination of beneficial bacteria work with certain foods like lignans to break down oestrogenic products in the intestines, binding the resultant molecules to food compounds and passing them down the intestine for excretion. The research findings that localised oestrogen is a factor in stomach, then colon, and thirdly rectal cancers makes the destruction of these good bacteria by antibiotics, chemotherapy drugs, steroids and the like particularly disturbing.

There are several strains of beneficial bacteria important to this process. You can only get *L.Shirota* in Yakult, but *L.acidophilus*, and *bifidobacteria* are available in pill form. Best are two 'multi-strain' pills: Prebiota 7, and Neways Advanced Probiotic.

Now that we live urban, sanitised lives, it is worthwhile taking these multi-strained supplements every day – but, as I said before, you have to feed them properly with whole foods, greens, grains and vegetables.

9. *Natural Progesterone*

Above I mentioned that foods like wild yam are known to limit oestrogen levels. One reason is that wild yam contains natural compounds that are the precursors of natural progesterone. And Natural Progesterone is a 'balancing hormone' for oestrogen.

It is important to understand that in research Natural Progesterone consistently comes through as a protective, life extending factor.

Synthetic progesterone – more correctly named progestin or progesten, is quite another thing – as the HRT studies have shown. Synthetic progesten has some uses in cancer treatment, but fundamentally the various HRT studies show it to be a dangerous and cancer risk increasing chemical.

Unfortunately studies into natural progesterone lag way behind the interest levels in oestrogen.

Natural Progesterone is not merely a 'balancer' to oestrogen, it is highly protective. For example, Guys Hospital conducted several studies in the mid- 1990's concluding that pre-menopausal women who had breast cancer operations during the second part of their cycle, when progesterone is highest, had twice the ten year survival rates of those who had the operation in the first two weeks of their cycle, when oestrogen dominates.

You may want to consider eating more natural wild yam as you age! Please beware a number of 'Natural Progesterone' products. Since they have been prepared and treated it is hard to understand how they are 'natural' anymore.

Summary

If doctors are going to give you anti-oestrogen drugs to 'prevent' a breast cancer returning, or a prostate from growing in size, then why not adopt an anti-oestrogen diet too?
The checklist includes:

- Be the right weight for your height.
- Cut your daily calorie consumption.
- Snack and graze – eat 6 small meals per day.
- Cut out sugar consumption.

- Cut saturated fats and trans fats – eat far more plants.
- Eat more phytoestrogens, like pulses, vegetables, greens, yams.
- Add resveratrol, quercitin, curcumin and indole-3-carbinol into your diet
- Only eat whole foods.
- Eat organic foods.
- Avoid toxic chemicals in the home.
- Drink clean water.
- Take asphalia (or melatonin) supplements.
- Supplement with beneficial bacteria daily.
- Exercise daily.

CHAPTER 20
EAT-TO-BEAT INFLAMMATION?

In 2000, the Mayo Clinic published results which showed that small daily amounts of aspirin would reduce the risk of prostate cancer by 40 per cent.

In February 2003 US scientists published a report in the medical journal, *Gastroenterology*, suggesting that aspirin cut risks of cancer of the gullet by 50 per cent.

In April 2003 there was a US desk study confirming daily aspirin prevents breast cancer.

In 2004 the Daily Mail ran the front page headline, '*Aspirin cuts Breast Cancer risk*'. Cancer Research UK were making news with research that showed 'an aspirin a day can slash the risk of developing breast cancer by almost a third'.

Aspirin was originally the active natural ingredient found in willow bark, and you can still find supplies.

One desperate truth about research on natural compounds is that it just doesn't receive anything like the exposure afforded to drug research by the PR machines of Pharmaceutical Companies, the Medical Authorities or even Governmental and Charity links. As a result expert scientists seem to be repeating the same fundamental pieces of research the world over, and the average oncologist and his hospital medical team knows little or nothing about it.

Herceptin will be front page news for months on end – another new study, this time with younger women; or a finding with a different cancer. Woe betide any health authority like NICE that dares to say the drug costs too much and they would rather spend their limited funds elsewhere. Dying patients who are 'denied' Herceptin are dragged onto yet more front pages.

Not so with natural compounds which cannot be patented and so can never be the source of pharmaceutical profit. Scientists the world over have proved and then confirmed several times over that certain foods reduce inflammation, and with it the risk of cancer. The research is then promptly forgotten!

Back in 2002, as I was writing an article on prostate cancer, I rang a UK charity for a view on the Mayo clinic's findings. The nurses on the 'helpline' had no knowledge of these findings saying that they did not like to recommend aspirin, and anyway the results were new and unconfirmed.

New??!! Unconfirmed??!!

26 years ago, in 1982, John Vane won a Nobel Prize and a knighthood for his work on **eicosanoids**. He was particularly interested in one group of eicosanoids called prostaglandins, which in excess can cause inflammation and concluded, even then, that they were reduced by aspirin.

Many experts, doctors included, believe hormones are made solely in the endocrine glands. In fact the largest volume of hormones in the body are the eicosanoids, very short-lived hormones lasting less than a couple of seconds at the most, and produced by the nuclear envelope of every cell in your body.

There are over a hundred and thirty known eicosanoids, each producing different responses; some helpful, some negative. Importantly, some eicosanoids, like prostoglandins, are helpful in small quantities but in excess cause significant problems around cells and in surrounding tissues, resulting in inflammation. Inflammation is a known precursor to many cancers.

Inflammation is more traditionally associated with conditions such as arthritis and drugs like Vioxx were created to tackle this.

These eicosanoids are the final and localised step in the communication process from your brain all the way to your cells. The messaging may be via any chemical – a hormone, a protein and even an electrical chemical. But put simplistically: Stressed brain, stressed breast cell. Happy brain, happy prostate cells.

Of course, the chemical that stimulates the local eicosanoid doesn't have to arrive under direction from your brain. A stressed breast cell could be the result of a number of other more 'random' chemicals too.

Inflammation – making bad eicosanoids

How are eicosanoids made? Basically all the fats and oils you eat, whether they are animal fats, fish oils, nut oils or fast food cooking oils are just a part of your body's oil pool, which we will call the 'fatty acid pool'. This pool provides the raw ingredients for the synthesis of all eicosanoids, 'good' or 'bad'. However, the production of bad eicosanoids requires an enzyme to cause the chemical chain reaction. This enzyme, called COX-2, is known, for example, to be stimulated by alcohol and fats in the intestine causing a carcinogenic bile acid, lithocholic acid, to be produced along with inflammation and the formation of polyps, and leading to colon cancer.

The COX-2 chemical pathway has also been shown to be stimulated by chemicals such as steroids, cortisol and insulin. So, science tells us that certain drugs, like **steroids**, commonly given to cancer patients when they are first diagnosed, can actually cause more inflammation at the cellular level. Large meals, high carbohydrate meals, excess sugar or sudden bursts of sweetened soft drinks or fruit juices will all cause **insulin** surges which stimulate the enzyme and turn the environment of your cells negative, significantly increasing the risk of cancer and other illnesses. And **cortisol,** the stress enzyme produced under direction from your brain by the adrenal glands, will also stimulate the enzymatic pathway producing more bad eicosanoids and inflammation. Cancer Research UK only recently in 2008 said that there was still no evidence that mental state and cancer were linked!

Diet – the good news

As various research studies have found, there are elements of your diet that can be highly protective. For example:

- The active ingredient of **aspirin** has been found in a number of studies to switch off COX-2, stopping it making 'bad' eicosanoids like prostaglandins. This same anti-inflammatory action would also be found in aloe vera which contains several such anti-inflammatory ingredients. Almonds will have a similar and natural analgesic effect.
- Long-chain **Omega 3** (found in fish oils) has also been shown to turn off COX-2 in a number of research studies from around the world.
- Ginger, **galangal** and **garlic** also contain ingredients that turn off the enzyme.

There is a small problem with aspirin. It doesn't seem to reduce inflammation in every case, just most cases. Andrew Chan of the Harvard Medical School (J. Nat Cancer Inst 2006. 98; 1494) believes that aspirin can play an important role in helping fight all cancers, but that the effectiveness may depend upon your genetics.

Vitamin D has been found to detoxify lithocholic acid (Howard Hayes Medical Unit, May 2002) and recent research has shown yet more natural compounds capable of reducing inflammation, notably the **phenols** in

- resveratrol
- olive oil
- green tea.

Finally, several US Cancer Centres are looking at curcumin as a way of reducing inflammation in colorectal cancers.

Eat-to-beat-inflammation

Most cancers go through an inflammatory stage first before becoming full blown cancer. This chapter started with breast cancer, but prostate would be equally relevant. The most well known inflammatory cancer is colon cancer, where inflammation produces polyps. Where colorectal cancer runs in families, regular monitoring to look for the development of pre-cancer polyps is 'officially' the standard practice in the UK. Sometimes, the doctor may suggest taking aspirin (the Mayo Clinic recommended 81 mgs). If you do, take no more that 100 mgs per day, always with food. Far better is to sip aloe vera last thing at night, or first thing in the morning on an empty stomach.

And then you can also take daily fish oils and eat far more oily fish in your diet. In the first half of the twentieth century UK fish oil production was regularly 75,000 tonnes per annum; now it is just 20,000. Sadly, we are consuming less fish and far less protective fish oils. (You can get short chain omega 3 from flaxseed and linseeds, but short chain is inert and only about 13 per cent converts in the body to long chain.) And you can always eat chopped raw garlic in your salads covered with olive oil, or you can steam food with grated ginger, washing it all down with highly protective organic red wine or green tea.

So eat-to-beat-inflammation? Easy. Fish oils, garlic, ginger, aloe vera, almonds, olive oil, curcumin, green tea and quite a few more natural anti-inflammatory foods and herbs. And even a glass of red wine!

CHAPTER 21
EAT-TO-BEAT INSULIN?

As we have seen, excess insulin can stimulate oestrogen production, IGF-1 production and 'bad' eicosanoid production – and each of these increases the risk of cancer. Insulin is also known to stimulate cell division and the prolonged exposure of cells to increased levels of insulin activates certain genes and changes their genetic behaviour.

Elevated blood insulin levels have been linked with increased risk of colorectal, pancreatic, liver, endometrial and breast cancers so far. Time will probably add to this list.

Then there is the fact that cancer cells have large numbers of insulin receptor sites on their surface, more than normal healthy cells. Cancer cells need lots of glucose and they need all the help they can get. Insulin brings the glucose to them. Research from Harvard comparing two matched samples of mice infected with cancer – one that had normal glucose metabolism, the other had the glucose metabolism blocked – showed that the group metabolising glucose all died, whereas 80 per cent of the blocked-glucose group survived the test period. Cancer cells love glucose.

So, insulin is implicated in cancer, as is glucose.

Diabetes

Diabetics have been shown to have an increased risk of cancer. For example in colorectal cancers that increased risk is threefold.

As I explained earlier, poor eating habits produce high levels of glucose in the blood. This in turn stimulates the hormone insulin to be produced. If you become diabetic, the problems do not stop. You may require insulin supplementation but the use of synthetic insulin is uneven during the day, with unused excesses at times.

The Medical Profession now understands the links between insulin and diabetes. They do not yet understand the relationship to cancer although the research exists.

So, an understanding of diabetes and factors that cause high insulin production is necessary both to help plan a healthy diet and to avoid cancer.

The source of insulin is the pancreas. Indeed, the pancreas makes two hormones: **insulin**, which takes excess sugar out of the bloodstream before it can reach and damage the brain, and stores it in the liver, muscles or fat cells, and **glucagon**, which responds to low blood sugar levels by causing stored glucose to be released. As we said earlier, a healthy liver is important to this process.

There are two common types of diabetes (although as many as eight different 'types' in all). Type 1 diabetes, which can be hereditary but can also occur after viral infection, sees permanent damage to the insulin producing cells in the pancreas and artificial insulin must be given to sufferers or they will go into a sugar-induced coma.

Type 2, or late onset diabetes, seems to occur typically when people are in their fifties and is usually the result of poor eating habits. However, it is not so 'late onset' these days with more and more adolescents and children succumbing to it.

For example, Mississippi is the worst region in the USA for late onset diabetes. In 2002 the levels had increased to 8 per cent of all adults. The health authorities blamed the high level of fried food and sweetened orange juice in the diet. Whilst in 1982 about 4 per cent of children (under 12s) in the USA had diabetes, by 1994 the figure had risen to 16 per cent!

The UK figures for diabetes are expected to double by 2010 (*British Journal of Community Nursing* 2002: 7). In the UK the growth rate of 'late onset' diabetes in under-fives is currently running at 11 per cent per annum (*BMJ* 1997: 315).

Late onset diabetes is diet related and had been simplistically linked to calorie intake. However it is increasingly thought to be caused by a complex mixture of a number of factors including high carbohydrate/sugar intake, being overweight, high intake of hydrogenated fats (i.e. trans fatty acids) and even milk consumption as we shall see.

The causes of diabetes – a modern diet

A French scientist, Dr Michel Montignac, developed a theory about the disease in the eighties which, although largely ignored at the time, is now generally believed correct.

Back in the seventies, scientists thought that all overweight people suffered from overproduction of insulin when ingesting carbohydrates, resulting in a storing of the sugars as fat. Montignac felt it was not obesity that was causing the diabetes but simply an overworked, exhausted pancreas.

By 1997 the Harvard School of Public Health had researched 65,000 women and concluded that the ones who developed diabetes most commonly ate a diet which was both low in fibre and also high in refined/empty sugars. (*JAMA* 1997: 277). A second study of 40,000 men supported this (*Diabetes Care* 1997: 20).

These findings caused a switch from the theory that a sedentary lifestyle, obesity and stress were causing the problems, pointing the finger of blame firmly at the intake of nutritionally 'empty' sugars and refined carbohydrate, i.e. a modern Western diet.

When the Harvard study also found that hydrogenated vegetable oils could bring on diabetes (*American Journal of Clinical Nutrition* 2001: 273) researchers started to understand why the disease was booming in the young. Hydrogenated vegetable oils are commonly used in fast foods and processed foods.

Another surprising contributor was then found to be cow's milk, which anyway contains insulin-like stimulators (IGF1) as we saw in a previous chapter. Finnish research (Diabetes 2000:49) concluded that children had a five-fold increase in diabetes if fed cow's milk during infancy. Mothers, your babies need to eat-to-beat-cancer too; breast is best!

Other factors linked to diabetes have been vaccines, beta-blockers and antidepressants like Prozac.

Interestingly the *Journal of Cardiovascular Risk* carried an article at the start of 2003 linking red wine consumption with protection against diabetes. No further comment from me is necessary!

The pancreas

The pancreas makes insulin and also produces pancreatic enzymes, which we have seen are thought by some experts to exert a controlling influence on cancer, by switching stem cells over to normal cells. If the pancreas is stressed by too much glucose in the blood stream causing endless demands for insulin production, it is possible that the pancreatic enzymes production line becomes stressed too.

This theory may well be borne out in reality. Research from the Mayo Clinic (Gastroenterology 2005) shows that elderly, late onset diabetes patients have an increased risk of pancreatic cancer.

The ingestion of refined carbohydrates and sugars

Sugar has been 'refined' for over two hundred years in an attempt to prevent it decomposing. It is now 96 per cent sucrose and can create a drug-like dependency in the body. Withdrawal symptoms are common in people who cut sugar from their diets. It also depletes the body of calcium. Corn syrup has similar problems and it depletes the body of B vitamins.

The average individual will consume over 170 lbs of sugar per year (Beasley, *The Betrayal of Health*). Processed and preserved foods are the main culprits as the sugar is hidden.

Our damaging eating habits are worsening. In the UK we start the day with our refined wheat, sugar-laced breakfast cereal (with added salt), and milk; then refined wheat toast and jams. You may even drink processed fruit juice (which is little more than sugared water anyway), and sugar in tea or coffee. In the USA there are refined grain waffles, hash browns and fried, calorie-heavy ham and eggs. The average American breakfast available at drive-ins for less than $7 is a killer. No wonder obesity is running at 26 per cent of US adults and its getting worse!

Snack food is sugar- and hydrogenated oil-rich. Consider empty calorie soft drinks, where a fizzy soft drink may contain ten spoonfuls of sugar; or chocolate, refined wheat bread, buns, cakes, pasta, ready meals, breakfast cereal, cheesecake and biscuits. Then you have an endless list of high street fast food outlets from burger to pizza 'restaurants'.

Natural fibre seems to have been forgotten in all this. Instead we take fibre supplements or enriched bran cereals. BUT. Natural cellular membrane fibre slows down the rate of release of sugar from <u>inside</u> those cells. Adding bran fibre to the diet on top of the other sugary foods cannot achieve this. It simply cannot stop the release of sugar from sugars!

Whole grains in our diet are also beneficial and protective in other ways. Many natural fibres, apart from aiding our excretion processes and bowel movements, contain compounds that can bind to and regulate fats in the bloodstream. As I told you earlier, high fibre foods are also the feeding blocks for beneficial bacteria in our guts.

Big meals, insulin rushes

It is not just the types of food that we eat that cause surges in insulin – it is the way we eat too.

As we said earlier, modern life means skipping meals and then eating just one or two big meals. Our hunger hormones will not quieten down until about 20 minutes after we start eating. By which time most hungry people will have consumed their whole plate full of calorie-rich, fatty and refined food. This causes great stress on the pancreas.

Glycaemic index

The refining process for grains, rice, processed meals and oils has a lot to answer for. Montignac went on to develop a diet or slimming plan. His basic recommendation was, "eat as much as you like but always foods with a **low glycaemic index (GI)**."

Sugar or glucose is the benchmark with a GI of 100. Refined foods which lack fibre, and over cooked foods, where the fibre (or cellulose walls of vegetables) has broken down, have GIs approaching 100 meaning a sudden rush of sugar into the bloodstream and an overworked pancreas. Foods like jasmine rice (109) or rice cakes (82) are typical of this. It is also why raw fruit and vegetables are so beneficial, as their intact fibre aids a slower and controlled sugar release process. All foods can be assigned a GI but this only measures their 'quality' in terms of sugar release. It needs to be coupled with their 'quantity'. Thus glycaemic load (which is what really troubles the pancreas) is the multiple of the two.

Thus spaghetti (150 gms) when cooked has 48 gms of

carbohydrate and a GI of 44. Hence the glycaemic load is 44 x 48 ÷ 100 = 21. So, when looking at the figures below, think also of the amounts you will consume.

Meats and fish have GIs of zero. Fresh, raw vegetables are usually 10 or below unless root crops. Fruits and nuts are usually in the 10–30 spread. Green vegetables around 15, pulses around 30.

Cooking takes carrots from 20 to 40.

GI foods – some examples:

Apple, raw	38	Muesli bar	61
Apple juice	40	Mung beans	39
Apricots, raw	57	Noodles, fresh	40
Apricots, dried	30	Oats	49
Banana, raw	52	Orange	42
Barley, boiled	25	Orange juice	53
Basmati white rice	58	Parsnips	97
Broad beans	79	Peach, fresh	42
Buckwheat, boiled	54	Peach, canned	58
Bulgar, boiled	48	Pear	38
Carrots, boiled	41	Pecans, raw	10
Chickpeas, boiled	28	Oat porridge, whole	55
Cereals, unrefined	40	Potato crisps	54
Cereals, refined	75	Raisins	64
Coco Pops	70	Rice noodles	40
Croissant	67	Ryvita	69
Fish fingers	38	Soya milk	36
Gluten-free muesli	39	Soya beans	14
Ice cream	65	Strawberries	40
Kidney beans	52	Sweetcorn	46
Kiwi fruit, raw	58	Sweet potato	44
Lentils, boiled	30	Wholemeal bread	71
Lychees, canned	79	Yam	37
Milk, fresh	31	Yoghurt, low fat	38
Millet, boiled	71		

It is interesting to note that the Bush people of the Kalahari and of Australia have their staple diet carbohydrates (e.g. Aboriginals use flour from the wattle seed) with GIs of only 10.

Low GI foods:

- Lead to lower insulin levels and rejuvenate a stressed pancreas.
- Help lower blood fats and cholesterol.
- Reduce risk of diabetes and heart disease.
- Reduce risk of cancer and improve overall health.

Eat-to-beat cancer?

You may wonder why I have suddenly started writing about diabetes. I don't want you to become diabetic, because it will increase your cancer risk. To summarise:

- Diabetes is linked with an increased risk of cancer.
- Poor sugar control leads to high sugar levels and causes pancreatic stress, increased insulin production and this leads to diabetes.
- Poor sugar control leads to high sugar levels and happy cancer cells.
- Excess insulin takes glucose to cancer cells. If you then become diabetic, the synthetic insulin can do just the same.
- Natural or synthetic insulin in excess can increase levels of oestrogen, bad eicosanoids and cell promoting IGF-1
- Type 2 diabetes is indicative of a poor diet – and low nourishment.
- Often type-2 diabetics are overweight, take limited exercise and carry toxins in their fat stores.
- A stressed pancreas may falter in its production of pancreatic enzymes thought by some experts to be crucial in controlling a cancer cell.
- Poor dietary foods reduce the excretion of toxins, and the levels of beneficial bacteria.

Can't lose weight – could this be insulin resistance?

There are an increasing number of serious studies in the USA about the inter-relationship of hormones in the cancer development process. Abdominal weight gain can often be a visible indicator of **insulin resistance,** and some estimates put the level of the population affected at 80 per cent. So you don't actually have to be in the 8 per cent of the population with diabetes, you may be in a more general 'insulin resistant' category. However it is still a result of poor modern diets.

Calorie Restriction

I've mentioned calorie restriction – and I will again later. Limiting calories – slows tumour growth and can even stop it. Indeed the various European studies have recently been confirmed by Harvard (Nova Science Now Jan 2007). They have even produced a video explaining how cutting your calorie intake by 30-40 per cent for any organism, can increase longevity by up to 60 per cent.

And the reasons they give are that calorie restriction:

- Reduces Insulin levels.
- Reduces metabolic rate and therefore toxin production.
- Increases the body's stress response, increasing survival hormones and strengthening the body's ability to control cell division and repair damaged DNA.

Summary

A simple finger prick blood test can show up insulin resistance. And a good nutritionist or naturopath can help you from there.
Meanwhile:

- Cut the empty calories, the refined foods, the processed foods and sugar from your diet.
- Graze. Don't eat just one or two big meals.
- Don't rely on 'added fibre'. Eat whole grain, and naturally fibre-rich foods. Eat more fresh and raw vegetables and fruit where the sugar is slowly released as the fibre breaks down.
- Cut bad fats and dairy from your diet.
- Take multi-strained probiotics.
- Eat more slowly. Take 20 minutes from starting to eat before the main course!
- Try and eat less calories than you need.
- Don't be overweight.

CHAPTER 22
OXYGENATING YOUR CELLS

Cancer thrives where oxygen is low

As I covered in the first section of this book, if you take a blood sample from a cancer patient and put it under a microscope you can usually observe two things: Firstly, the white, immune system cells are 'lifeless' whereas in normal blood they move around. This is a sign that your immune system is impaired. Secondly, the red cells are often clumped together – a sign that both iron and oxygen-carrying levels are low.

Cancer cells use lots of iron and they thrive when oxygen conditions are low.

In 1931, Otto Warburg won a Nobel Prize for this discovery that cancer cells didn't use oxygen – in fact it could kill them.

Since then, German and American scientists have pioneered treatments which aim to get oxygen into cancer cells. Hence the 'alternative' therapies, which use ozone to try to oxygenate the cells, or high doses of vitamin C, or hydrogen peroxide and glutathione as pre-oxidants to get inside the cell and bring about increased oxygen levels.

Warburg himself concluded that the best way to fight cancer was to get oxygen to the cancer cells and to do this you needed highly oxygenated blood in the arteries (as is normally the case) but also highly oxygenated blood in the veins (normally very low in oxygen) to create a 'bottleneck' and a cellular oxygen overload. This is easier said than done. Since veins carry about 70 per cent of the body's blood volume, (arteries carry about 17 per cent, with about 13 per cent inside the organs), you have to somehow get oxygen into vessels that are returning from the organs and tissues immediately they exit the tumour area. The theory of tissue 'oxygen overload' has taxed some of the world's best cancer specialists for the last 70 years.

Certain factors work against cellular oxygen levels. As we have said before, high levels of oestrogen or high sodium levels can both reduce cellular oxygen.

Depression limits blood oxygen; and depressed people develop more cancers.

Indoors, outdoors

Many people reading this will immediately think of their external environment. Do I live in fresh air near trees and mountains or do I live in pollution, near a main road or factory chimney?

In Chapter 2 I told you that The US Environmental Protection Agency stated in 2006 that indoor air is two to five times more polluted than outdoor air on average, citing 1,500 hazardous substances in the average US home. Typically these include airborne pollutants from household cleaning products, and personal care products, second hand smoke, radon, formaldehyde from pressed wood products, biological agents such as fungi, mites and bacteria and nitrogen oxide from gas appliances. The EPA went on to say that the air in some homes could be 25 to 100 times more polluted than the air outside, and that airborne indoor pollutants from cleaning and personal care products are three times more likely to cause cancer than pollutants outside.

We also use in-house pesticides from plant sprays to medicated shampoos and mosquito repellants. For example, carbonates have been linked to increased levels of child leukaemia (Insern, France); and in-home insecticides containing chlorpyrifos have been affecting testosterone levels (Epidemiology Jan 2006). Not surprisingly, women who stay at home have 40 per cent more toxins in their blood than their identical sisters who go out to work. After all, they have laws governing toxins in the work-place, but at home you are free to pollute your environment as much as you wish. Concerned readers should go to our web site and read an article entitled 'As safe as houses'.

Never allow anybody to smoke in your home. The biggest direct hazard to our blood oxygen is smoking, with its carbon monoxide level, which blocks the haemoglobin oxygen-carrying sites. Passive smokers have been shown to be six times more threatened than was originally thought and women are twice as prone to the damaging effects of smoke as negative airway factors have been found to be carried by the X chromosome – women have two X chromosomes, men just one (Cancer

Research UK). Children are particularly at risk in homes where a parent smokes.

Polluted air doesn't stop with cigarette smoke. A number of toxins in the air we breathe make us vulnerable to cancer. Motor vehicles emit hazardous toxic chemicals, which collect on dust particles – and we breathe these in. People living near main roads, children living near garage forecourts, both have increased rates of cancer. Sunlight can encourage these polluted dust particles to become even more toxic, making Nice on a bad day almost three times worse than London.

These particles collect in the deepest recesses of your lungs and are virtually impossible to clear out. This results in increased levels of toxins in the bloodstream, with further toxins collecting in body fat and organs like the kidneys. Diesel fumes have been noted as the third largest cause of lung cancer in the USA.

Polluted, sunny cities can also have oxygen levels as low as 12 per cent on a bad day compared with the 21 per cent of air normally attributed to oxygen. At 7 per cent life ceases. The US Environmental Agency reports that over a hundred million tonnes of various toxic chemicals are released into the atmosphere every year in the USA. The Nation (September 17 1990) reported that autopsies on one hundred young people in the Los Angeles region showed that all had lungs suffering from toxic air pollution damage.

Increasing your blood oxygen – breathe, eat, exercise

Breathe: Get to the hills! Get outside where there really is clean, fresh bracing air. And walk, briskly if possible; breathe. An important part of Chinese cancer treatment is deep breathing exercise.

The fact is that most of us do not breathe properly. Unless we do something strenuous we tend only to use the top third of our lung capacities, allowing toxic air to sit and stagnate at the bottom of our lungs. This prevents toxins moving out of our bloodstreams and into our lungs to be excreted. Moreover, deep breathing moves the lymph in the thoracic duct and this can increase the lymph flow throughout the whole body, pulling toxins away from the cells.

Eat: Correct iron levels will help too, and many foods, especially green vegetables, are excellent sources of readily assimilated organic iron. They will help you carry more oxygen in your blood stream especially if you live in an outdoor and sunny environment. Russian research on chlorophyll (including chlorella and spirulina algae) has shown the molecule to be very similar to the haemoglobin molecule. One argument put forward is that a good consumption of 'greens' doesn't just provide cancer fighting elements like iron and vitamin K, the action of sunlight combined with the chlorophyll actually increases blood oxygen levels, through photosynthesis. Some people argue that this is why people in the US 'sunbelt' tend to get less cancer – because they are farmers with higher vegetable consumption. Some cancer experts are trying to use this theory in a treatment called Photo-Dynamic Therapy.

People with higher blood glutathione levels are 'healthier' according to several research studies. This is especially true for older people. You can increase glutathione levels by a diet rich in green vegetables and fruits – especially organic ones. Glutathione helps the mitochondrial power stations of your cells incorporate oxygen.

Exercise: Medical science has proven conclusively that fit people are ill less. And fit people recover quicker after an illness or an operation.

The magazine 'Integrative Cancer Therapies' in America reviewed all their research studies where cancer patients had taken exercise and concluded that people with cancer who did daily exercise had 50 per cent less mortality.

Researchers at the University of Bristol have conducted an extensive review of 52 international studies on exercise and found that physical activity can significantly reduce the risk of cancer, and improve the chances of survival if you do have it. From 37 of the 52 studies on exercise and breast cancer incidence, scientists found evidence that showed typically a 30 per cent reduction in the risk of the disease in women who exercised on a regular basis. Generally, the benefits of exercise were stronger for post-menopausal women than pre-menopausal women.

A 2008 study of girls and young women who exercise regularly shows that those who do, cut their risk of breast cancer before the age of 50 by almost a quarter. High levels of exercise between the ages of 12 and 22 offered the most protection. It is thought that exercise reduces oestrogen levels as well. It is quite worrying then, that in a UK report in February 2003, 20 per cent of school children now do not do any exercise in the average week.

There are many more studies, mainly from the USA. The most important conclusions are that:

- Exercise helps prevent cancer.
- Exercise helps survival.
- The exercise does not have to be strenuous.
- But it does have to be 'daily' – ideally for about 30 minutes.

For example, in 2003 researchers at Fred Hutchinson Cancer Research Center, Seattle, showed that exercise did not have to be strenuous. Women who exercised a little, but every day, reduced their risk of breast cancer 17 per cent. There is even research that shows that physically active people, housework and making the beds included, reduces colon cancer risk by 22 per cent.

Finally, all manner of exercise types can be useful. For example The Center for Integrative Medicine, Thomas Jefferson University Hospital, Philadelphia, studied cortisol levels amongst over 10,000 people. Typically in stressed situations, the brain stimulates the adrenals to produce cortisol, and I have told you that this can cause cellular inflammation, a precursor to cancer. A doctor might tell you to go home and rest. Researchers found resting would reduce cortisol levels just 5 per cent, whereas your first ever yoga class reduced levels nearly 25 per cent.

Taking 'exercise'

The Government Health Authority's official recommendation is that you should take 20 minutes exercise three times per week. If you want to beat cancer, this advice is undoubtedly wrong.

Another problem is that many people find it all too stressful to think about gyms. And there are a number of reasons for this:

The 'losing weight' myth: Firstly, too many people set goals of weight loss for their new-found exercise routines. This is not the prime reason to exercise. You are doing it to be healthier – reducing certain dangerous hormone levels, moving your lymph, oxygenating your blood etc.

Next people seem to expect to lose weight quickly and set unrealistic goals anyway. One pound of fat contains approximately 3000 calories. Your first hour on the bicycle in the gym will burn around 400 calories if you can pedal for that long!

Also you will start to put on a little muscle – this is a good thing, but muscle weighs more than fat so no wonder the pounds don't fall off you at the start! However, over the weeks as you rebuild some lost muscle, an upward spiral starts. For every pound of muscle you add to your body, you burn 30 calories per day just to maintain it. So by losing three pounds of fat and gaining three pounds of muscle you might feel gloomy when you stand on the scales, but over a week the extra muscle will be burning a 1000 calories or so, even when you have a day off and are sitting watching the TV. Given the daily recommended intake for a woman of 1500–1800 calories and a man at 2200–2800 calories you can see that the benefits will start to grow. Stick at it. Bear in mind that we are not talking about building 'muscles', just converting some of the fat back into the state it was, in your youth.

Many women may be daunted by images of being surrounded by lycra-clad young lovelies 'going for the burn'. Be reassured. Too much exercise produces even more toxins in the body, burns up certain vitamins and is increasingly thought to be counter-productive. This is part of the reason why so many top athletes are so often ill or end up with diabetes.

So stop worrying – do not think, *'Exercise to lose weight'*. Think, *'Exercise for health'*. All those happy hormones produced, less oestrogen, more oxygenated blood, less depressed etc.

Exercise for health should simply be a sensible, controlled and long-term commitment to a healthier you. *"Never confuse motion with action"*, as Ernest Hemingway said. You may see much motion down the gym but the best regimes are planned action programmes for health, not slimming.

The crucial issue is to better understand what you should try to achieve in your fitness programme and weight loss is simply not the number one priority – it will come over time.

i) Oxygenate your cells

Most fitness books talk about the benefits to your heart and circulatory systems and it is true that you should see a gradual improvement in your blood pressure and your peripheral cardio-vascular system. Your heart will become stronger and your blood more oxygenated. This is one of the biggest goals in your plan to beat cancer.

Your lungs will learn to work again. Blood passing past a lung that is using 100 per cent of its capacity will be able to clear out more toxins. In turn it will become more oxygenated.

As the blood system strengthens it will carry this oxygen to the most distant cells much more efficiently than before.

ii) Move your lymph

You have twice as much lymph in your body as you have blood. It bathes the cells and is supposed to transport wastes and toxins away from the cell, and then to transfer them to the blood stream for excretion. The only problem is that the lymph system has no heart to move it away from the cells and pump it round the body. When you sleep at night, your whole lymph system 'sleeps'. Only you can get it moving again in the morning!

The largest lymph duct is the thoracic duct, which passes across your chest. You must move your lymph daily to clear toxins away from your cells. And you must replace it with clean lymph, which is where exercise and clean water enter the equation.

Yes, of course your lymph will be moved if you take exercise. But other less strenuous pursuits will do the job just as well. Deep breathing and stretching will affect the thoracic duct. Light yoga exercises and graceful Tai Chi. And swimming and press ups of course. Even yawning and laughing help move the lymph across the chest.

Exercise will also improve your posture, which in turn helps remove restrictions on your lymph and energy flow.

As your peripheral circulation improves, so too will your peripheral lymph system allowing the toxins to move out of even the most distant cells. Massage can also help with this lymphatic drainage.

iii) Everyday movement

The basic rule with fitness is to 'think active' – try to be active every day in your normal life. In one study, a group of Chinese people were found to be burning 3500 calories per week in 'natural' exercise. That's the equivalent of one hour on the bike in the gym every day! But then, US research in Epidemiology magazine says that the women with the lowest risk of breast cancer are those taking 6 or more hours of exercise per week. By all means go to the health club for professional advice, but on your days off try yoga, do deep breathing, walk the dog, have a swim. Build your own personal programme of activity. Recent research showed that women who make the beds every day have less colon cancer! Be active in your everyday life. It will pay dividends

iv) Have fun

Working out oxygenates the blood, and low blood oxygen is associated with depression. Exercise also produces endorphins, often called happy hormones. These are addictive – you will increasingly feel more energised, happy, less stressed and lighter in spirit. Endorphins neutralise stress hormones like cortisol and so can change the environment of even your breast and prostate cells, through eicosanoid production as we discussed. There is some evidence that they decrease levels of oestrogen as well. Active exercise helps the biochemical environment of every cell in your body. It's illogical to spend lots of money on chemical antioxidants and toxin-free products if at the same time you allow your cells to float in stressed, toxic surroundings.

v) Boost your hormones

Yes, you may decide you want to lift some weights in the gym. Lifting weights to a point of having tired muscles will cause Human Growth Hormone (Hgh) to be produced. If you are over

50 years of age you are hardly making this hormone any more, but resistance training will produce a shot of growth hormone at almost any age.

Hgh is a powerful neutraliser of free radicals, and helps to further eliminate fatty deposits and builds lean muscle. In research studies in America with Hgh, people over 50 reported regaining lean muscle mass, losing fat and feeling youthful and re-vitalised. It helps men and women avoid osteoporosis too, without the need for supplements like HRT.

vi) Health and happiness, not slimming

Please understand that you are making a commitment for life. It's not about instant weight loss, it is about overall health and well-being: Moving your lymph, oxygenating your blood, building more muscle tone, increasing the good and happy hormones and, eventually, after 3 to 6 months, sure, you may shed some fat. But please don't go near the scales for three months!

Some days you may go to the gym with your new friends, others you may do yoga in your front room, or walk the dog, or swim, or simply have a massage. Allow yourself a little constructive pampering every now and again!

Drink plenty of water after your exercise to flush out those toxins, and eat protein within two hours of the work out to rebuild the muscle.

Action?

Take the first step!

If you want to prevent cancer, and certainly if you have it already, it is crucial you give serious consideration to where you live, your in-home environment and how to get a good source of quality oxygen into your lungs on a regular basis.

- Do not smoke, do not have people in your home who smoke.
- Use toxin-free household products, personal products and avoid toxic sprays.
- Do not live near main roads or sources of diesel fumes.
- Live well away from factories or other sources of air pollution.
- Learn to use your lungs and breathe properly.

217

- Eat plenty of green vegetables.
- Be active: Take daily exercise.

CHAPTER 23
EAT-TO-BEAT YEASTS AND MICROBES

Most people reading this book have a parasite

In my book, *Everything You Need to Know to Help You Beat Cancer*, I covered the view from the World Health Organisation that 20 per cent of cancers are caused by infection. Some experts think this figure is low. Parasites do not have to be three feet long. They can be microscopic like the ones in Carolina that come in the household drinking water as they have become immune to chlorine. Parasites can come with sushi, overseas travel, exotic fruits and even kissing (mucky habit!) The term parasites can also include viruses, bacteria and yeast infections.

Several factors are common. They all deplete you of your nourishment – they do live off your body, after all. And they can produce toxins, some of which may be carcinogenic. And sometimes they can also create unfavourable conditions inside tissues, for example, leading to a lack of oxygen.

- Increasingly, parasites are felt to have a link to cancer. In one study 42 out of 1000 patients in a USA cancer hospital were found to have a liver fluke. This was eradicated and many treated patients recovered. Fluke in British livestock has increased four-fold since 1997.
- Some parasites can produce known carcinogens like aflatoxins.
- 17 cancers are already known to be caused by viruses. As detection methods become more refined who knows how many the final total will be?
- More and more evidence is being produced on the role of a bacterium, *Helicobacter pylori,* in stomach cancers. This bacterium 'hides' from the acid in the stomach by diving into the mucous membrane. This causes the immune system to rush to the other side of the lining, setting up the conditions for an ulcer. In extreme cases of inflammation and in the presence of localised oestrogen a cancer can form.

219

- Excessive yeast populations are thought to be present in 70 per cent of the UK population, and are often living pretty much undetected. *Candida Albicans* is the main culprit. You may have thrush, or cystitis. Or bloating after meals and wind. Typically, males may have yellow toe nails.
- In a case history in America a nurse 'with leukaemia' was cured simply by killing her yeasts. 27 per cent of her child leukaemia ward then achieved the same 'cure'.
- Many 'parasites' simply drain the immune system as it constantly tries to eject them or nullify their toxins. Many parasites are associated with a depletion of B vitamins. Several B vitamins are crucial for their role in the cancer process: As I told you, biotin boosts the immune system, choline and inositol help de-fat the liver and folic acid is vital for accurate DNA replication.

Many parasites can be detected by a blood test or a stool analysis but the lab technician will only look for those parasites he has been told to look for, so things do get missed. Microbe, virus, bacteria and yeast detection can also be undertaken by 'Alternative' practitioners who use analytical systems like VEGA. Nutritionists, herbalists and homeopaths can then help you work to eradicate these unwelcome polluters. In Germany the use of such 'alternative' systems is far more commonplace than in the UK and is available on the state health service to all patients. In the USA many more people go for parasite checks than do in the UK. In Japan many people take daily anti-parasite supplements (raw fish is a common and increasing source of parasites).

Yeast Infections

US research concluded that women who had had 25 'doses' or more of antibiotics in their lifetimes had double the risk of breast cancer. Researchers decided to go and look at how antibiotics might affect breast tissue.

Another study in the US showed that taking daily cinnamon supplementation could reduce the symptoms of type 2 diabetes in 25 per cent of cases. Researchers decided to go and look at how cinnamon interfaced with insulin and glucose.

Oh dear. Why not talk to a good nutritionist instead. They will tell you what is going on: In one word the problem is, 'Yeasts'.

As we saw in Chapter 15, antibiotics kill bacteria. Not just your infectious ones, but even the beneficial ones in your gut. At night, one of the prime roles of beneficial bacteria is to protect you by devouring the yeasts and microbes you consumed along with your food during the day. One estimate I read said that in a healthy individual the 'friendly' bacteria could devour up to two pounds of these yeasts and microbes a night!

If they are not present in the right quantities, the yeasts and microbes start to multiply uncontrolled. This can result in all manner of gut problems from Irritable Bowel Syndrome (IBS) to Crohn's, ulcers and even cancers.

Also, yeasts are like mushrooms – they can form colonies and take root, making holes in the gut wall, causing leaky gut. An excess of yeasts can cause toxins in the blood stream making you inexplicably tired, increasing food allergies and far worse. Sometimes yeasts can also cross in to the blood stream from where they may pass to an area of the body and colonise it. Yeasts are anaerobes – they do not use oxygen to 'live'. So they create a whole non-oxygen world. Your healthy cells may then be deprived of oxygen. You might expect them to die, but no, they just adapt to metabolise in the absence of oxygen. And this is called a cancer cell.

Now, not every cancer cell or every cancer is 'caused' in this way. As I keep saying – the causes of your cancer can be many and can be as individual as you are. But I am not surprised that antibiotics would be linked to higher rates of cancer – it makes perfect sense. And I'm sure that if the 'experts' checked the figures for other drugs; they might find some similar statistics.

Some yeasts move round the blood stream and stick, using a little carbohydrate, to the surface of cells. Unfortunately this blocks the cells' ability to receive important messages via surface receptor sites. Some of these sites may be insulin receptor sites. So this makes it harder for insulin to remove sugar from the blood stream and it will appear to be failing – and this may be confused with the effects of diabetes. However, it is widely known in hot climates that cinnamon kills yeasts in the blood stream, thus reducing the cell surface blockages and allowing some supposed diabetes sufferers to get sugar out of their blood streams into the cells. One wonders why the 'experts' haven't worked this out too.

Indeed, if you go round the world and look at the warmer countries where yeasts would be more prevalent you see that there have lots of natural foods that protect the populations. The following all kill off yeasts via their daily consumption: **Garlic, chilli, bee propolis, caprylic acid** (coconut), **cinnamon, nutmeg, fennel/anise, oregano, Pau D'Arco** (South American tree bark) etc.

The problem in the UK is that we simply do not consume anti-yeast foods any more. And we reduce the numbers of beneficial bacteria in our bodies by caesarian birth, not breast feeding, no longer living on farms, chlorinated water, stress, antibiotics, drugs, pasteurised foods and so on. No wonder 70 per cent of our population has excess yeasts.

If you have a yeast infection you must address it.

In the last few years I have visited a number of specialist cancer clinics. In every case, I always go and talk to the people at the 'sharp end', the nurses!

What has astounded me is that they have all been adamant that every cancer patient they treat has a bad yeast infection – women and men. But this should be public knowledge. Back in 1993 *Contemporary Oncology*, a major cancer magazine for doctors in the USA, stated clearly that people suffering from cancer who had radiotherapy and or chemotherapy did not die from their cancers *"but finally succumbed to an infestation of candida albicans"* (**common yeasts!**).

Yeast 'poisoning'

Perhaps the best way of thinking of 'yeasts' and similar 'infections' is to regard them as microbes. Yeast infection is microbial infection.

Yeasts may be thought of a little as you would 'fire' – fire is helpful to humans in a controlled form, but devastating if allowed to get out of control. Gerald Green is the grandson of Professor Fritz Haber who discovered how microorganisms fix nitrogen leading to an understanding of a number of substances from fertilisers to explosives. Gerald is extremely knowledgeable about such microbes himself and I am indebted to him for increasing my knowledge.

If you have an excess of yeasts in your body, apart from feasting on the nutrients your body and immune system needs, they will create waste products. Some of these are mildly toxic and will reduce your immune defences further. But also *candida* microbes produce an 'alcohol'. This poisons the bloodstream, making you feel 'hung over' and lethargic, and invoking serious work from your liver to detoxify it. Even worse, it feeds the cancer cells. **This alcohol produces a by-product and cancer cells thrive on it.**

As I covered in Chapter 15, the real breakthrough of the last 5 years has been a much better understanding of the role of beneficial bacteria and their interrelationship with food, and microbes in your body's health systems.

For example, we know that *Helicobacter pylori* is a bacterium that causes stomach cancer. It can be treated, although not perfectly, by a combination of three antibiotic drugs – or you can use the herb **Goldenseal** with **bismuth** and **acidophilus**, along with a protein diet (no carbohydrate) to increase stomach acid which normally kills it. A little aloe vera, sipped slowly first thing in the morning and last thing at night will help calm the inflammation as will fish oils.

Recent research has shown that the phenol compounds in both **Extra Virgin Olive oil** and in **Green Tea** can both prevent and treat *Helicobacter pylori*. Apparently they can still operate in the stomach's acid and were effective even when antibiotics were not. Other studies from the USA show that **curcumin** can kill the bacterium *in situ*.

There are several parasite and yeast 'killers'. **Pau D'Arco** is very effective; in fact it was originally thought to be a cancer killer. But the best parasite and yeast killer is probably a natural Chinese herb called **Wormwood**. It has proven more highly effective than drugs against malaria too.

A company called Neways makes a product called **Parafree** which will see off most parasites – the course lasts two months and you and your partner both need to do it (as I said, parasites can be passed by kissing). Parafree contains all natural remedies like black walnut, pumpkin seed, garlic, anise, butternut, fig, clove, ginger and pomegranate seed.

So, when did you last eat raw honey, fennel, pumpkin and its seed, cloves, oregano or pomegranate – all popular in England 500 years ago?

Eat-to-beat yeasts

There is an effective anti-yeast diet which involves:

- Consuming no sugar in any form (lactose, dextrose, glucose, honey etc).
- Consuming no dairy.
- Consuming no alcohol.
- Consuming no yeast products like marmite and mushrooms.
- Consuming no fruit save on an empty stomach first thing in the morning, and never after a meal.
- Consuming no 'soft' vegetables like marrows, cucumbers, squash or courgettes. Both groups can sit on top of the food in the stomach and ferment.
- Taking Pau D'Arco, Caprylic Acid, Garlic, Wormwood, oregano and cinnamon, and topping up with multi-strain probiotics.

Junk foods, fast foods, branded fruit juices, processed foods and foods from crisps to breakfast cereals are to be avoided as they often contain both yeasts and sugars. Go fresh and home cooked!

When attempting an anti-candida diet, expert Gerald Green recommends participants avoid certain carbohydrates too, especially refined carbohydrate as this can turn to sugar. For example, he recommends avoiding:

- Bread and all relatives.
- Cereals, hot or cold.
- All snack products from crisps to popcorn.
- All white rice, potatoes, corn and refined wheat products like pasta.
- Most fruit.

- Root vegetables.
- Lentils, chickpeas, dried beans.
- All coffee, caffeine, fizzy soft drinks, fruit juices, alcohol.
- All convenience/junk foods.
- All cows' dairy.
- All processed meat products (bacon, sausages, salami).
- All high salt foods.
- All mushrooms and fungi.
- All condiments.
- All hydrogenated fatty acids and saturated fats.
- Health supplements containing lactose, gluten and citric acid.

His good food choices include:

- Alfalfa and sprouting seeds
- Sweet peppers
- Broccoli, Brussel sprouts, cauliflower, cabbage and greens, kale, chard
- Endive, fennel, garlic, onions, spring onions
- Green beans
- Hot chilli peppers
- Lettuce, spinach
- Parsley
- Radishes
- Olive oil, flaxseed oil, fish oil
- Eight glasses of water per day
- Herb teas
- Whole oats, psyllium seeds
- Free range eggs
- Fresh fish
- Pork, lamb, veal
- Chicken, turkey, game
- Quorn, soya milk, rice milk, sheep's and goat's milk
- Soda bread (wheat free) with no added sugar or salt.

For your information, fresh garlic, when you cut it, oozes like a fresh potato. It does not have a green stem in the middle, nor does it appear as concentric leaves like an onion. It doesn't smell and it is hot on the stomach. Two cloves a day uncooked would be good. (If you buy the 'leafy' variety in your supermarket, you should know that taking the green centre out avoids the stale 'garlic' smell.)

Gerald recommends Pau D'Arco and Wormwood, plus half a teaspoonful of freshly ground cinnamon in a glass of water. It helps fight the *candida* in the bloodstream, reduces sugar levels and stops the microbes forming the alcohol used by the cancer cells. (N.B. Patients with Type 1 diabetes must not use this).

Homeopaths have nosodes (natural potions that stimulate disease responses) to treat yeasts and these too can be very helpful.

And, when you undergo your 'yeast cleanse', you must also aim to strengthen your immune system. The following could be helpful:

- Vitamin C with bioflavenoids: 5 times per day 200 mgs each time
- Vitamin E: total 8 forms, 400 IU
- Zinc: 15 mgs
- Selenium: 200 micrograms yeast-free
- Chlorella

The herbs echinacea and astragalus are also recommended.

If you do need to sweeten things, use Stevia. It is a natural leaf sweetener and apart from being considerably sweeter than sugar it has antifungal and anti-bacterial properties. (Stevia can be obtained in the USA but is not on general sale in the UK – it is frowned upon by the sugar cartel.)

certain natural compounds have the ability to repair damages already occurring in healthy DNA – this could have incredible importance, not least to patients having radiotherapy and chemotherapy. Hopefully one day your doctor will have the knowledge to tell you exactly how you can keep your healthy cells from damage when he is trying to kill the cancer cells.

But the sad truth is that whether it comes to killing the germ, or to nourishing the terrain we have lost our way in the UK. We just do not eat these natural compounds in the volumes we did, or should do. And it is no surprise, in my opinion, to see our cancer rates and five-year survival figures well below average in Europe.

So here is a selection of natural compounds you might like to include in your weekly menu. Some are 'Natural Foods' and others are 'Natural Compounds'. I have just chosen an indicative 20. It could have been 100. Well, for example, there are over 4,000 plant, vegetables and fruits containing flavenoids already identified! What is relevant is that often the 'active ingredient' is the pigment – the metabolite that confers part of the plant's natural colour. Bees seem to know this. Their hives and honey are full of natural compounds from the colourful pigments that attracted them. So if you want to be healthy, you need to accumulate these colourful natural pigments in your diets too!

Anthocyanins

Background: Dr Ferenczi may have cured himself and a number of patients with his beetroot diet because beetroot contains anthocyanins and these are known cancer cell killers. Typically these compounds are blue in alkaline and deep red in colour in acidic conditions and are formed from anthocyanidins and their precursors pro-anthocyanins, usually in combination with various sugar molecules. There are a great many anthocyanins and they have many different functions for the plant. They are antioxidants, protect the plant against UV-light, are a defense mechanism and are very important in pollination and reproduction, attracting insects.

Sources: the main sources of anthocyanins are beetroot, blackcurrants, dark olives, elderberry, figs, deep red plums, red grapes, blueberries, blackberries and some vegetables, such as aubergine, red onion, red cabbage, avocado and hawthorn. The volume in certain fruits, especially if organic, can be 1-2 grams per kilo.

Eat-to-beat cancer benefits: Used as a staple in Russian soup, beetroot and these other foods have antioxidant properties. Anthocyanins have been the subject of many experiments – there are more than 200 articles in PubMed on the benefits of anthocyanins. Benefits include:

- They seem to provide protection to the DNA.
- They reduce the growth rate of cancer cells, and tumours.
- They have anti-oestrogen activity.
- They have anti-inflammatory benefits.
- They increase white cell levels and stimulate the immune system.
- They inhibit cancer enzymes and can directly kill cancer cells (apoptosis). For example, researchers at Ohio State University have shown that eating these purple foods slowed the rate of growth of colon cancer and actually killed up to 20 per cent of the cancer cells.

The biggest problem is that research is difficult because they seem to interact so freely with other plant compounds. Also, like quercitin, these plant compounds are broken down extremely rapidly in the body making it hard to follow all the various metabolites and what they are up to!

Oligomeric Proanthocyanidins (OPC's)

Information: OPC's are very powerful antioxidants, reportedly 20-50 times more powerful than vitamin E. They scavenge and neutralise free-radicals. Much work is being undertaken with these products and cancer, although they already have other known benefits and effects, for example:

- Heart and blood vessels – in artherosclerosis, high blood pressure, high cholesterol and poor circulation and varicose veins.

- Limit complications occurring due to diabetes – e.g. macular degeneration, eye and nerve problems.
- Wound healing.
- May inhibit destruction of collagen.
- May thin the blood and so may double up with drugs trying to achieve the same ends – be careful.

Sources: Commonly found in Grape Seed Extract and Pine Bark in slightly different forms. Proanthocyanins are also found in tea, red wine, cranberries, apples and pears. Pycnogenol (from French Maritime Pine Bark) is highly promoted in the USA.

Eat-to-beat cancer benefits: The US National Cancer Institute records a number of anti-cancer studies including:
- Breast and prostate cancer prevention.
- Reduction of damage to breast tissue after radiotherapy.

Ellagic Acid

Information: Ellagic acid is an extremely stable polyphenol. Dr Daniel Nixon at the Hollings Cancer Institute, at the Medical University of South Carolina (MUSC) began studying ellagic acid in 1993. It is a proven antioxidant, anti-carcinogen, anti-mutagen and anti-cancer initiator.

Sources: It is found in some 46 different fruits and nuts, for example pomegranate, red raspberries, blackberries, strawberries, blueberries, cranberries, pecans and walnuts.

Eat-to-beat cancer benefits: Ellagic acid is a proven anti-cancer agent. Initial studies and clinical tests have shown that ellagic acid can protect the *p53* gene. Recent published data from MUSC includes the findings that:
- Ellagic acid has anti-bacterial and anti-viral properties.
- It can prevent HPV infected cells developing, and cervical cells infected with HPV experience apoptosis (normal cell death).
- It slows the growth of abnormal colon cells. It increases the rate of metabolism of carcinogens and prevents the development of cancer cells.

- It affects and inhibits the action of acrylamides, known as potent carcinogens. And, as a powerful antioxidant, it neutralises the affects of aflatoxins produced by parasites within the body.

And all this seems to come from eating just **half of one cup of red raspberries per day!**

Resveratrol

Background: Resveratrol is the exciting new kid on the block. It is a phenol and comes in two forms cis- and trans-. Both forms are found in the skins of a number of fruits and plants, where its prime function is to protect against potential invaders like moulds and fungi. One benefit of resveratrol, is that it can stimulate the hormones (Sirutins) that are stimulated to protect the body when on a calorie restricted diet. Sirutins are linked with longevity. Pharmaceutical companies are trying to synthesise compounds that can achieve the same result.

Sources: Typically, red grapes and red wine – especially organic varieties, as pesticides kill the moulds and fungi that cause its promotion. Much smaller amounts (about 10 per cent of these levels) also occur in blueberries and bilberries and even smaller amounts in raspberries and blackberries.

Eat-to-beat cancer benefits: A great deal of new research:
- Fights yeast and fungal growth.
- Resveratrol seems to also stop tumour growth (maybe due to calorie restriction/sirutin promotion since that effect is also linked to stopping tumour growth.)
- Protects DNA, repairs DNA.
- Reinstates action of the p53 gene.
- Kills cancer cells.
- Prevents metastasis.
- Anti-inflammatory.
- Seems, in research, to be potent with difficult cancers such as gliomas and prostate.

A 'Wonder Compound' – both a preventative and chemotherapy agent (MD Anderson Cancer Center, Texas).

Pterostilbene

Information: There is little research on this natural compound as yet – but what there is seems extremely promising. It is an aromatic hydrocarbon and a derivative of resveratrol. It was originally praised for its anti-fungal and glucose-lowering benefits. US Department of Agriculture researchers have found that it acts in a similar way to the drug cipofibrate, using cellular receptors to lower LDL cholesterol and triglycerides. However, unlike the drug, it has no side effects of muscle pain and nausea.

Sources: It is part of the blue pigment in blueberries, cranberries, loganberries, and grapes. It was originally isolated from Red Sandalwood.

Eat-to-beat cancer benefits: Rutgers University and the US Dept. of Agriculture have said that the compound is a powerful antioxidant and seems to mop up free radicals especially those that lead to polyps and colon cancer. Further work by Agnes Rimando at Oxford MS and at The Uni. Of Med. Sciences Poznan, Poland has shown a cancer cell killing ability with breast cancer, plus an ability to turn off an enzyme called cytochrome p450. Cytochrome P450 enzymes activate a variety of compounds known as "procarcinogens", which can turn substances such as cigarette smoke and pesticides into carcinogens. Hence pterostilbene seems to be a great protector.

Curcumin

Background: The active 'ingredient' of the orange/brown spice turmeric. It inhibits bacterial action in the intestine and stomach, it is an anti-inflammatory, boosts cellular glutathione levels, is a powerful antioxidant, and can prevent and treat cancer. American cancer centres have done a lot of work on curcumin in the last three years.

Sources: A member of the ginger family, it has been used in

Ayurvedic medicine for years. Levels to obtain benefit are way in excess of those you would achieve by having a few curries though!

Eat-to-beat cancer benefits:
- MD Anderson says it can prevent and treat cancer.
- Tufts have obtained results with breast cancer, using curcumin and isoflavenoids to limit environmental damage,
- Kentucky University say it inhibits leukaemia cells
- Sloan-Kettering used green tea spiked with curcumin and concluded it was a cancer beater – it prevents tumour formation and stops the development of the essential blood supply.

There are a dozen or more studies where it causes cancer cell death and even more where it prevents tumours forming a blood supply.

Green Tea

Information: Green tea contains polyphenols, which the lack of processing leaves unaltered, while the drying process concentrates. Polyphenols are powerful antioxidants, protect against heart disease, lower 'bad' fat LDL levels and stop artery plaque building. You need to exceed 10 cups per day for the full benefits. Some of the polyphenols, called catchetins are 5 times more potent than vitamin E. They help in limiting diabetes effects, and green tea even helps in weight loss (University of Geneva).

Sources: India and Asia – *camellia sinensis.*

Eat-to-beat cancer benefits:
- One catchetin in green tea (EGCG) has been shown to be effective against UV induced skin cancer.
- It can also inhibit the spread of cancer (Nature 1997, Jankun).
- EGCG has been shown to limit oesophagael cancer even amongst smokers and drinkers, by 60 per cent (Shanghai).
- EGCG has been shown to block an enzyme that multiplies cancer cells, causing their death.
- It also promotes beneficial bacteria in the intestine.
- The Mayo Clinic claimed their research showed 4-7 cups per

day could 'stop leukaemia in its tracks'!
- Research from Perth shows drinking one cup per day reduces ovarian risk by 60 per cent and prostate risk by 33 per cent.

There are studies on colon, breast, prostate and other cancer, and even studies that show it enhances radiotherapy and chemotherapy, whilst reducing side effects.

Olive Oil

Information: Olive oil also contains polyphenols. And extra Virgin Olive oil seems to be particularly 'healthy'.

Eat-to-beat cancer benefits:
- The Journal of Agriculture and Food Chemistry 2007, covered research on how Extra Virgin Olive Oil can both prevent and treat *Helicobacter pylori* infections.
- Olive oil polyphenols have also been shown to reduce inflammation by inhibiting COX-2.
- The University of Ulster have shown another ingredient, oleocanthal is particularly important in reducing inflammation.
- Danish scientists have shown that olive oil reduces oxidative damage to cells.

Chaparral

Information: A Native American evergreen desert shrub, long used by Native Americans to treat everything from colds to infections, and even skin cancers.

Eat-to-beat cancer: The usual method is to make a tea or poultice. The University of South Carolina has shown that Chaparral does indeed have the ability to shrink some tumours. Despite warnings from the FDA that this could cause liver and kidney damage, researchers have now started to inject a refined extract M4N into patients with head and neck cancers, seeing results where orthodox treatments had failed. Cancer Research UK have said that clinical trials on M4N will be important.

Capsaicin

Information: One of the active ingredients in spicy peppers. One of a number of compounds called vanilloids. Already used in the treatment of muscle strain and psoriasis.

Sources: Chillis

Eat-to-beat cancer benefits:
- Research indicates that the natural compound can kill microbes in the stomach.
- It is also effective against certain types of skin lesions and skin cancer.
- 2007 research by Nottingham University showed that this natural compound could actually knock out an enzyme which is unique to the power production system of a cancer cell, and is not found in healthy cells. Scientists are hoping to prepare a drug based on this compound.

Indole-3-Carbinol

Information: In 2004/5 the pharmaceutical company Hoechst started to patent indole-3-carbinol (I3C) and a number of its close relatives. It claimed that eventually these new compounds will be used to treat all manner of illnesses from arthritis, to MS to cancer, and even replace Tamoxifen with a better alternative. I3C is a member of the glucosinolates family. This family contains other indoles and also isothiocyanates such as sulphoraphane.

Sources: Indole-3-glucosinolate is found in broccoli, kale, cabbage, bok choi, Brussel sprouts, cauliflower and turnip. Upon chopping or mastication it releases I3C.

Eat-to-beat cancer benefits: It works at a number of levels (and it may not actually be the I3C that is working but by-products following breakdown in the intestine).
- An antioxidant, neutralises free radicals.
- Inhibits Human Papilloma Virus (HPV).

- Inhibits certain aflatoxins, and revents aflatoxin-induced liver cancer, leukaemia and colon cancer.
- Liver protector.
- Stops cancer cells growing and increases death rate of cancer cells.
- Restores p21 gene preventing synthesis of DNA for new cancer cells.
- Reduces and even reverses oestrogen driven cancers
- By blocking oestrogen sites on cell membranes
- By converting highly active oestrogen variants into safer sisters
- By blocking other cancer enhancing receptor sites
- By directly killing cancer cells.

It has been dubbed (by UCLA and others) the 'safer, natural Tamoxifen'- it inhibits breast cancer cell proliferation by 90 per cent, whilst Tamoxifen scores 60. I3C also neutralises the by-products of oestradiol breakdown, whereas Tamoxifen has no effect.

UCLA and Strang have shown that it can have a big effect on neutralising attack from chemicals such as oestrogen mimics and dioxins, and their dangerous breakdown products.

The average daily Japanese consumption level is 120 mgs per day. And research studies usually use 200-400 mgs. Some people are sensitive to this substance. Some people have a genetic mutation preventing some of its actions.

Sulphoraphane

Information: Sulphur compounds play an important part in blocking cancer cell formation. Garlic's active compounds are sulphur based. Sulphoraphanes are indoles – see I3C.

Sources: Brassica and broccoli. And especially sprouting seeds.

Eat-to-beat cancer benefits: Research has shown that sulphoraphane (SUL) can inhibit the development of breast cancer cells. Research covered in Proceedings of the National Academy Oct 2007, showed that sulphoraphane activates cancer fighting enzymes inside the skin to fight melanoma and skin cancers. The researchers used broccoli seed extract. Several other cancers are being studied.

Garlic

Information: Garlic crops up time and time again in the fight against cancer, whether we are looking at Asian diets, or Mediterranean diets, glycoproteins or yeast control. The bad news is that **fresh, chopped or squeezed garlic is essential.** Cooking ruins the effect and, in tests, some garlic pills are pretty useless. There are several active ingredients. Most garlics have active sulphur ingredients. Although many reports talk about the active ingredient being allicin, other anti-cancer agents appear to be produced on cutting or crushing. Other ingredients include alliin and the enzyme allinase.

Eat-to-beat cancer benefits: Garlic has strong anti-cancer benifits.

- It seems to restrict the blood supply to cancer tumours and thus stops them growing.
- Garlic is particularly protective in stomach, gastric and colon cancers and, across several epidemiological studies, it has been linked to reduced rates of a wider range of cancers, from lung to oesophageal. For example, in the Iowa Women's Health Study (USA Steinmetz 1994) of 127 foods, tested with 41,387 women, garlic was the only fruit or vegetable that produced an effect; one or more servings of fresh garlic a week was linked with 35 per cent less colon cancer and 50 per cent less distal colon cancer.
- In a 1998 study in China (You et al) people taking large quantities of garlic every day (up to 60 gms per day!) had less than half the cancers of those taking only a little.
- It is possible that allicin works as an antioxidant, and it is certainly effective in reducing blood cholesterol levels. Allicin is also a very strong natural weapon against microbial infection, particularly bacteria, viruses, yeasts and intestinal amoeba. Allicin interferes with enzymes necessary for the growth of these microbes and also enhances a liver enzyme, which detoxifies aflatoxins before they cause damage. Allicin

thus wards off infection and allows the body's natural defences to be stronger.

- Allinase seems to promote this action and in tests, allicin has been shown to inhibit cancers of the breast, liver and colon.
- Allicin appears to bind to breast cell receptor sites preventing the action of cancer agents. Prostate cells exposed to the garlic chemical SAMC grow at only 25 per cent of the normal rate.
- Garlic also seems to protect the body against the side effects of radiotherapy, particularly DNA and chromosome damage.
- Professor Wargovich of the University of Texas has been working with two other active ingredients: dialylsuphide and S-allyl-cysteine. These have been shown to reduce animal cancers by 50 to 75 per cent and, in another test on animal cells, to totally protect against a deliberate attempt to induce a particularly virulent oesophageal cancer.
- Some garlics contain good levels of selenium and these varieties have been particularly successful in treating breast cancers. Garlic is anyway a good source of glycoprotein polysaccharides.
- Garlic also contains good levels of tryptophan, which is the precursor of serotonin, which in turn is the precursor of melatonin. Melatonin, as we saw earlier, is an excellent and very powerful neutraliser of free radicals.

Fish oils

Information: Dr Benjamin Frank (*Nucleic Acid Therapy in Ageing and Degenerative Disease*) showed, nearly thirty years ago, that we need to produce about one to one and a half grams daily of nucleic acid. Dr Frank believed that nucleic acid rich foods could retard or even reverse the ageing process.

Top of his list was fish, which he believed should be eaten at least seven times per week. He also suggested freshly made fruit or vegetable juice and good water intake. Apparently **all** his patients benefited from his diet.

Fish oils have been proven to aid general body health, preventing heart disease and dementia, increasing IQ's in children and also to aid cancer prevention and control.

The origins of these long-chain polyunsaturated fats are the microscopic algae and plankton that the fish feed on. Sadly, of course, fish farming methods may mean less consumption of these vital nutrients. This is why the best fish is 'deep-sea caught'.

Eat-to-beat cancer benefits: Fish oils contain omega 3, vitamin A and vitamin D, and most contain good levels of selenium and some vitamin E. They also contain long-chain omega 3 which is known to reduce inflammation in tissues. These have all been shown to have very active roles in beating cancer. Thousands of years ago we consumed one unit of omega 3 for every unit of omega 6, 9 and others in total. Now a New York twenty something consumes just one unit for 50 of the other oils. But your body really needs it. Research shows that omega 6 can actually accelerate the growth of human prostate tumours. (Cancer Research UK). Omega 3 can balance this.

Inflammation, especially in colon cancer, depends on the enzyme COX-2. Levels of the enzyme are high in 85 per cent of colon cancers (Dubois, Vanderbilt), and also in breast cancer. Work is underway on drugs, which block COX-2. **But why take drugs when the fundamental answer lies in increasing your intake of fish oils?** The *International Journal of Cancer* (March 2002) reports on 250 women with breast cancer and the findings that **women who are cancer free have much higher omega 3 fatty acid levels in their breast tissue!**

Polysaccharides, or glycoproteins

Information: Four Nobel Prizes for Medicine in recent years (1994, 1999, 2000 and 2001) have been won with research on how cells communicate, and the importance to our health and well-being.

Three had implications for cancer prevention and treatment.

In 1994 Gilman and Rodbell won for their discovery of 'G-proteins and how cells handle signal substances from glands, nerves and other tissues to make changes.

In 1999 Gunter Blöbel and his team looked at how proteins have specific protein signals built into them so that they reach the correct destinations.

And by 2001 Hartwell, Hunt and Nurse had won for showing

an understanding on the cellular messages involved in the cell cycle – its growth and division into two identical daughter cells – and how mistakes might result in a cancer development.

Blöbel also found out why your immune cells could not recognise some cancer cells – and it was all to do with imperfect membrane structures then being stuck to by carbohydrate molecules.

These protein messages often involve complex sugars, and so it is common in the USA to call them 'supercarbs' or monosaccharides (which is actually wrong as most are polysaccharides). In fact most are a combination of 'sugars' and peptides (small proteins of less than 30 amino acids in length). You can't make these sugar chains – and nor can you break them.

Sources: Aloe vera; arabinogalactins (found in carrots, leeks, radishes, corn, pears, red wine, coconut meat, tomatoes, curcumin and echinacea); brans (slow cooked oatmeal, whole barley, brown rice); breast milk; garlic; pectins (apples, pears and citrus fruit eaten whole). Shiitake mushrooms contain 1:3 beta-glucan polysaccharide and medicinal mushrooms in general are strong suppliers of polysaccharides (reishi, cordyceps, maiitake, shiitake); psyllium seeds. MGN-3 (or Biobran) is made from rice bran and enzymes from shiitake mushrooms. It is one of the most powerful immunomodulators currently available. Breast milk is another big source of glycoproteins – nourishing brain cells and boosting the immune system in babies.

Eat-to-beat cancer benefits: Even very small amounts can make a big difference. Eat the right polysaccharides and they will help clean up your membranes, stop the carbohydrates sticking and the immune system can spot the good, the bad and the ugly and will itself be greatly boosted. Pharmaceutical Companies are working on drugs to enhance this process – you can eat the foods.

One polysaccharide complex is being used in branded supplements by a major health company and is recommended by 'Alternative' cancer experts. The basis of the complex supplement is simply D-Mannose – and you can buy a natural source D-Mannose, by going to our website.

Professor Gilbon-Garber has shown that the invasive process of bacteria, viruses and indeed cancer cells which involves the above 'bonding' process to membranes, can be inhibited by glycoproteins in mother's milk. Because these molecules used in her experiments are all-natural, no side effects occurred. Many experts believe that the discovery of polysaccharides could turn out to be more important than vitamin C or antibiotics.

Nitrilosides

Information: There are at least 1,200 species of plants in the world that are nitrilosidic and the natural compounds are often described as nitrilosides or beta-cyano-genetic glucosides. Sadly in the UK we are eating less and less of those that were indigenous to us like gooseberries, blackberries, blackcurrants, quince, millet, maize, barley, watercress and pulses.

Sources: Flaxseed, linseed; bamboo shoots, grains: barley, buckwheat, maize, millet, blackberries, black and redcurrants, cassava, cranberries, gooseberries, loganberries, quince, raspberries, strawberries, yams, papaya; brown rice, pulses: lentils and many pulses like kidney beans and fava beans. Nuts: For example, pecan nuts, macadamia nuts, cashews, walnuts, almonds. Beans: For example, lima beans and field beans; sprouts like alfalfa or Mung bean; watercress, sweet potato. The seeds of lemons, limes, cherries, apples, apricots, prunes, plums and pears.

Eat-to-beat cancer benefits: There is a group of approximately 14 compounds which are water-soluble and are dubbed vitamin B-17 or amygdalin. B-17 has been used as a cancer treatment for a number of years. Amygdalin was first isolated in 1830 and used as an anti-cancer agent in Russia as early as 1845. But it was reborn by the father/son team Ernst Krebs senior and junior, who isolated a purified form of the active ingredient (calling it laetrile) and, with others in the late fifties to seventies, sought to explain its action.

Cancer cells differ in a number of ways from normal cells. One difference as we have said earlier is that the mitochondria, or power stations, do not use oxygen to produce energy, and need a whole different energy system and a different set of chemicals (enzymes). In a cancer cell there is a unique enzyme called glucosidase which breaks down B-17 into hydrogen cyanide (which kills it) and benzaldehyde (an analgesic). In normal cells, where glucosidase is virtually non-existent, another enzyme, rhodinase, renders the B-17 harmless. Critics talk about B-17 containing cyanide but, as we have seen so far in this book, hundreds, if not thousands, of plant compounds can 'contain cyanide'. Proponents clearly believe B-17 is a seek and destroy missile targeting only the cancer cell mitochondria.

Well, maybe. Every day you produce several hundred cancer cells. Get them early with a rich B-17 diet and this could be true. However, as cancers develop they often form protective protein coats around the cells to ward off the immune system. These protein coats will protect the tumours from B-17 too.

Various cancer clinics have thus developed 'metabolic therapy packages'; these include bromelain (from pineapple), papain (from papaya) and two pancreatic enzymes trypsin and chymotrypsin to break down this protein coat, plus vitamins A, E and B complex, plus high dose vitamin C and high dose minerals.

The difficulty then becomes, "which bit worked?" Having personally talked to leading B-17 therapy users in the USA and Europe, none doubts its efficacy, but all felt it was not as potent as high dose vitamin C or pancreatic enzymes and that clearly a significant contribution was being made by the other participants in the therapy package.

Laetrile is the synthetic form of B-17 and has shown effectiveness against cancer cells *in vitro*, and in rats and mice. Even the NCI, which is negative about laetrile, reports that by the late seventies over 70,000 cancer patients had been treated with laetrile and there are copious case histories on its effectiveness. Dr Contreras of the Oasis of Hope Hospital in Mexico is one of the foremost advocates of B-17 therapy. He has dubbed it 'nature's chemotherapy', and uses it on all cancer treatments but notes that it does not work for brain tumours, sarcomas or liver cancer.

Krebs recommended eating ten apricot seeds per day for life as a preventative measure (the seeds, or kernels, have the highest levels of B-17); cancer treatments use four to six 500 mg tablets per day or intravenous injections.

One issue is overdosing as cancer patients most usually have toxic livers, and an enzyme, glucorinide, in the liver will have to detoxify any excess B-17. **A maximum of five kernels at any one time in a two-hour period is recommended for preventers or cancer patients,** and cancer treatments have to be properly super-vised. I met a gentleman in Australia who had prostate cancer and had been to a speech on B-17. He was taking 50 kernels for breakfast and wondered why he felt sluggish and livery!! Excess B-17 and cyanide by-products have been known to build up in the liver. Each of us has different liver detoxing capacities and the cancer patient has an already impaired liver. Cyanide poisoning of the liver can result if excess is consumed by someone with an impaired liver. **1 gm of vitamin B-17 is the maximum recom-mended dose to be taken at any one time and the US Nutrition Almanac recommends a maximum of 35 seeds per day.**

Genistein, red clover and soya

Information: Isoflavones are widely found all over the world in herbs, plants and vegetables being an alternative term for flavenoids. Flavenoids have been shown to exhibit a number of anti-cancer benefits in research.

- With Colorectal cancer (Italy).
- With Laryngeal cancer (Italy).
- With Ovarian cancer (Washington University).
- With Breast cancer (Greece/USA).

Some of them have oestrogenic power – phytoestrogens, are similar but not identical in chemical composition to oestrogen; however their action in the human body is much, much weaker than the human hormone and as such they have been dubbed protective and even called 'anti-oestrogens'.

Isoflavones and phytoestrogens have been very protective to people in the UK for thousands of years. Red clover, the herb of Hippocrates, has a long history of use as a medicinal herb. It's an excellent blood purifier that gradually cleanses the bloodstream and corrects deficiencies in the circulatory system. It is found as a central ingredient in a number of herbal anti-cancer formulas, including the Hoxsey formula, Jason Winter's tea, and Essiac tea.

Sources: Flavenoids are abundant in plants, vegetables, fruits, herbs and pulses. Typically many people talk about phytoestrogens in pulses like broad beans, peas, flageolet and lentils; or chickpeas and hummus; or in red clover.

Eat-to-beat cancer benefits: There is a lot of mythology and argument. Several US 'experts' and even the FDA had dismissed red clover as useless in dealing with cancer. Some even think it dangerous. Red clover contains four main oestrogenic isoflavones, daidzein and genistein and compounds called coumestans, for example, biochanin and formononetin.

- Red clover is being studied with breast cancer patients at the Royal Marsden.
- Researchers at the National Cancer Institute have confirmed that there are indeed anti-tumour properties in red clover.
- Georgetown University in Washington, DC have found that genistein increases repair protein levels in the cell, and this helps prevent damaged messages being passed on. These repair proteins are regulated by genes such as the BRCA genes and only low levels of repair proteins are usually found in cancer cells.
- According to the NCI, genistein has the ability to prevent tumours from developing the blood supplies they need to survive, thus starving and killing them.
- Genistein, like other phytoestrogens, has also been shown to have the ability to block receptor sites on cells preventing the much more active human oestrogens like oestradiol binding there. Genistein is used by Plaskett in his therapy and by a number of clinics to treat hormonally driven cancers.

Genistein levels in red clover are about ten times the level found in soya. Little of the other active ingredients are found in soya.

Pulses formed an important part of the UK diet 100 years ago but no more. Pulses do contain protein and oils and these are frowned on by the more extreme cancer therapies, like Gerson, where even modest levels of fat and protein are forbidden. Pulses can also contain phytic acid, which prevents the absorption of certain minerals. Fortunately this rises to the surface on boiling and can be skimmed off.

Soya is an incomplete protein and lacks vitamin B-12. Fermented soya products have a less effective anti-oestrogenic action. Some mass-market soya milks are GM originated. You should also beware of mass-market soy sauces as they have high sugar and salt content. Shoyu and Tamari, brewed in oak casks are more natural but still high in salt, albeit sea salt.

Cancer Research UK contributed to a study which looked at soya consumption and cancer in Eastern women. Women who consumed the highest amounts had 60 per cent fewer cancers than those who ate the least.

Asian women, who have far, far less cancers than Western women, have up to a thousand times the isoflavone levels in their bloodstreams when compared to their Western equivalents, and many studies have concluded that this is a vital and protective factor.

Citrus isoflavones are being used with limited success for brain tumour treatment, isoflavones have been shown in small scale studies to aid the effectiveness of radiotherapy.

Chlorella and spirulina

Information: The earliest life forms; over 30,000 species inhabit the earth where there is a natural water supply. At one extreme are microscopic blue-green algae, at the other 150 foot long strands of kelp.

Probably the best known are spirulina and chlorella, both having many properties in common, although unlike other algae chlorella has a nucleus.

They are excellent sources of vitamins and minerals, enzymes (including digestive enzymes) and amino acids (with all eight essential acids). However, they have notable other benefits.

Eat-to-beat cancer benefits: Spirulina and chlorella are both excellent sources of polysaccharides. Chlorella contains mannose, arabinose and galactose amongst others. These help communication between cells and your immune system to identify rogue cells.

A large number of Japanese studies have shown how both boost white immune cell levels – interferon and particularly T-cells.

Chlorella seems to enhance levels of lactobacillus in the gut aiding the immune system and general nourishment.

Both have excellent levels of beta-carotene (about ten times the level of carrots), organic iron and vitamins D and K. In chlorella, B vitamin levels are excellent, especially B-12, although folate levels are low.

Chlorella helps in detox diets since it can help bind heavy metals and some pesticides, supported by the action of intestinal bacteria, making elimination easier.

The interesting development, though, is in the use of such chlorophyll-rich algae as agents in photodynamic therapy. Russian work shows that the chlorophyll, which produces oxygen when light is shone on it, can destroy cancer cells and US research (Waladkami, Clemens, 1990) has shown how important green vegetables and phytochemicals are in the restriction of cancer development.

There is an increasing body of opinion that chlorophyll (which has a similar molecular structure to haemoglobin) can circulate in the bloodstream and even help to oxygenate (and kill off) cancer cells by photosynthetic action. The sun belt that runs through the USA is also the area where people have the highest vegetable intake, and the lowest cancer rates.

Quercitin

Information: Another flavenoid, it is also a phytoestrogen and features in both the Gerson and Plaskett therapies and is increasingly being shown in research to have many benefits. Quercitin is metabolised very quickly in the intestines and liver after ingestion and very little is found in the blood. This has greatly hindered research to date. Now more studies are looking at the effect of its metabolites. One hypothesis is that even small doses are very important to humans, and the speed of its metabolism and destruction was no problem because quercitin is so widespread in fruit and vegetables – 100 years ago we ate fruit and vegetables all the time continually 'topping up' the levels of quercitin.

Sources: Commonly apples, onions and tea. But also (in descending order of concentration) capers, the herb lovage, red grapes, citrus fruits, rhubarb, green vegetables including broccoli, cherries, raspberries, chokeberries, and in small amounts in tomatoes and honey.

Eat-to-beat cancer benefits:
• Specifically it is an antioxidant, an anti-histamine and an anti-inflammatory agent.
• It has also been found to be an effective 'hyperthermia sensitiser'. Hyperthermia can kill cancer cells.
• UCLA research found that quercitin used in conjunction with ultrasound can effectively kill both human prostate cells, and skin cancer cells (*British Journal of Cancer* (2005) 92, 499-502).
• This makes it a potential adjunct in the treatment of various cancers that are sensitive to heat stress or hyperthermia (e.g. leukaemia, colon, prostate, melanoma etc). Its formula is related to the group of compounds called anthocyanins.
• The Mayo Clinic report that their research shows that quercitin blocks the androgen pathways in prostate cancer, slowing or stopping prostate cancer cell growth. They believe quercitin could provide a non-hormonal alternative to prostate cancer therapy. (March 2001)
• Research by the Italian Cancer League has shown that it prevents the growth of prostate cancer cells. And the skin of apples has been shown to inhibit colon cancer.
• It stops the proliferation of cancer cells in vitro, especially if vitamin C is present (Kandaswami).
• Quercetin and genistein are the most potent anti-proliferating flavenoids in colon cancer (Kuo).
• Quercetin has potential in the treatment of leukaemia (Teofil).
• Quercitin is a phytoestrogen and there are two studies suggest-

ing positive effects with breast cancer and lung cancer, but these need confirmation.

• The University of Maryland and the Cedars-Sinai Centre report that quercitin flavenoids seem to enhance several chemotherapy drugs, but may be themselves damaged by chemotherapy drugs. They can also have the same effect as certain antibiotics. Whether this means there is a clash with antibiotics, and quercitin should not be taken at the same time, or it actually enhances the antibiotic effect is not fully understood yet.

Bee propolis

Information: Bee propolis has always had a pretty healthy image. After all, honey was one of the staple foods in the Middle Ages and is known to have significant anti-viral and anti-fungal benefits. Propolis is a natural compound produced by bees from the buds of plants and mixed with wax and resin. It is used to repair the hive, and to protect it from predators like viruses, bacteria, fungi and various microbes and diseases. It maintains the temperature and health of the hive (Park et al 2002).

Not surprisingly, it can be extremely useful in fighting various infectious diseases. A range of safe and positive effects has been identified – for example, it is highly effective with:

• Wound healing.
• Skin infections.
• Tissue repair.
• Gastro-intestinal problems.

The actual content of bee propolis depends on the geographic location of the bees and the time of year (Banskota et al 2000). Propolis often comprises more than **180 natural compounds, many of which are concentrates of powerful antioxidant plant flavenoids and phenols.** The bees seem to understand the importance of The Rainbow Diet! Bee propolis is now also known to have:

• Anaesthetic benefits
• Immuno-modulating benefits

- Anti-inflammatory benefits
- Antioxidant benefits
- Cardiovascular benefits
- Cancer prevention and treatment benefits

Sources: Brazilian bee propolis (Green propolis from Baccharis Dracunculifolia) has been the subject of many serious clinical studies, and according to PubMed, accounts for over 26 per cent of all new research. Because the 'ingredients' of bee propolis can vary greatly, I will confine the rest of this piece to Brazilian green propolis. (Much of the research detail comes from an article published in the *International Journal of Cancer Research 3 (1); 43-53 2007*).

Eat-to-beat cancer benefits: Brazilian bee propolis has significant and varied anti-cancer benefits, some of which will surprise many orthodox experts. Furthermore, it has been shown to enhance the benefits of chemotherapy and radiotherapy, having a protective effect on healthy cells and an enhancing effect on chemotherapy action.

(i) **Anti-inflammatory action**
Propolis has been shown to inhibit prostaglandin, leucotrine and histamine release (Khayyal et al 1993; Mirzoeva and Calder 1996; Hepsen et al 1999). In each case the response was as good as the recommended prescription drug (Menezes et al 1999). Propolis was even found to overcome formaldehyde induced arthritis. Typical active ingredients were the flavenoid hesperidins (Hata and Beyer 2004).

(ii) **Anti-viral; anti-yeast**
Various research studies have confirmed bee propolis effectiveness against all the principle strains of *Staphylococcus, Escherichia coli, salmonella, E coli, candida albicans* and even *HIV*. A number of flavenoids seem particularly important, especially kaempferol, pinocembrin and galangine. Controls were taken using prescription drugs such as AZT the anti-AIDS drug. Moronic acid

in propolis had significant anti-HIV effect, out-scoring the AZT drug.

(iii) **Wound healing**

Propolis has been found to have antiseptic, anaesthetic and healing powers. It has been shown to have a healing effect in the tissue repair of oral mucosa (Bretz et al 1998) – hence the use of Manuka by Christie Hospital, Manchester for patients after orthodox therapies with mouth or throat problems. It is also effective as a 5 per cent mouthwash after dental surgery (Carvahlo 1994). Post operative wounds – for example after cancer surgery – in subcutaneous tissues were more quickly healed with a compress of propolis, honey and comfrey ointment (Magro-Filho 1987).

(iv) **Immune stimulant**

The ester of caffeic acid (CAPE) is one of the main active compound of propolis, along with the flavenoid ingredients quercitin and hesperidine. They seem to have two actions. Firstly, they seem to inhibit cellular growth and secondly, they can increase the presence of certain white immune cells like T-lymphocytes, increasing hydrogen peroxide production without any simultaneous and damaging nitrite production, which usually occurs with macrophage activity. (Than et al 2003; Ansorge et al 2003)

(v) **Free radical scavenging**

The many flavenoids give propolis its powerful antioxidant benefits. Matsushige et al 1996 isolated a compound from propolis to show that it had a stronger antioxidant benefit that vitamins C and E.

(vi) **DNA protection**

CAPE, even when used in low doses, can prevent cellular mistakes in healthy cells and induce apoptosis (cell death) in cancer cells. Thus it seems to have a double benefit of protecting healthy cells whilst killing cancer cells. (Chen et al 2003). This selective effect was previously shown by Su et al in 1995.

(vii) Anti-tumour effect

The ability to protect healthy DNA was confirmed by Banskota et al 2001, and by Suzuki et al, in 2002. They both also noted that propolis had anti-tumour activity. The ability to kill cancer cells has been shown both *in vitro* and in animal *in vivo* studies. The particular ingredient responsible is Artepillin C, which leads to cancer cells' DNA fragmentation (Kimoto et al 1998). Kimoto has also shown that intra-tumoural injections of 500 mgs of Artepillin C produced apoptosis and an increase in immune defences.

CAPE and another 20 ingredients of propolis were tested by Nagaoka et al 2002. 4 were found to cause cancer cell death. Where CAPE was taken orally by mice with lung tumours, a reduction of tumour size of 50 per cent was noted. Researchers similarly tested another group of mice using the drug cisplatine. No difference in effectiveness was noted, but the mice taking the drug had significant weight loss, a side-effect not noted with propolis (Nagaoka et al 2003). It was concluded that CAPE had a cytoxic effect, and could also block the invasive metastasis noted with these tumours.

(viii) Enhancement of orthodox chemotherapy approaches

Propolis has biological effects that act in synergy with chemotherapy drugs such as 5-fluorouracil (Suzuki et al 2002)

Importantly, Santos and Cruz 2001 showed that the antioxidant properties of propolis could reduce the side effects caused by chemotherapy drugs without any detriment to the therapeutic effects.

Suzuki researched two drugs in experiments with mice and cancer (mitomicine C and 5- fluoresce) and showed that the combination of drug plus propolis had by far the greatest regression effects especially in advanced stages, over the drugs used on their own. The propolis usage resulted in higher levels of white and red cells and less side effects. The conclusion of the research was that propolis increased the bio-availability of the drugs. The desired effect could therefore logically be achieved on smaller doses and with even less side effects.

Orsolic and Basic (2005) used mice with breast tumours to show antioxidants can enhance the performance of both radiotherapy and chemotherapy, by using water soluble bee propolis. This supports the work of Chan, noted above, that CAPE has a cytoxic effect and can cause cell death, whilst protecting the DNA of healthy cells. 'Chemotherapy agents used in anti-metastatic activity have their benefits enhanced' was again the conclusion. The authors recommended clinical trials should take place as all the indications were for greater effect in radio and chemotherapy, whilst minimising blood cell declines and other side effects.

Padmavathi et al (2005) studied the drug paclitaxel with propolis, in DMBA-induced mice breast cancer and concluded that the two in combination suppressed breast cancer, decreased lipid peroxidation, and increased the activities of antioxidant enhanced super oxide dismutase and vitamin C. They concluded that the combination of paclitaxel and propolis offers maximum effect in DMBA-induced breast cancer.

Overall

I have provided an extended look at bee propolis.

Firstly, because it is a 'super-concentrate' of a **rainbow diet** of natural compounds. The bees have done it for you. It is what this book is all about. They have partaken of 180 natural compounds from all manner of plants whose pigments and colour attracted them.

Secondly, because, yet again, these natural compounds have research that shows they can provide wonderful health benefits.

Thirdly, because it can help you beat cancer.

Fourthly, because it can increase the effectiveness of radiotherapy and chemotherapy, whilst reducing the side effects and protecting healthy cells. Something too many oncologists in the UK deny is possible.

Eat-to-'beat cancer?

Now, do you believe me? Adding these natural compounds into your diet, in a way that they can combine synergistically and enhance the effects of each other is going to increasingly be shown as the way our diets worked 200 years ago. Then we ate honey, and herbs like parsley, sage, rosemary and thyme, and lovage and feverfew. And basic vegetables like turnips, beetroot, watercress, cabbage, broccoli, sprouts, peas, broad beans, tomatoes, potatoes, parsnips and carrots. And fruits like apples, pears, quince and black and red currants, gooseberries and berries from the hedgerows.

This 'rainbow' diet of colours protected us and nourished us – and is unrecognisable to the great majority of teenagers in 2008.

CHAPTER 25
EAT-TO-BOOST YOUR
IMMUNE SYSTEM

How do I boost my immune system?

It is one of the most asked questions of our charity staff. People who want to prevent disease know that a strong immune system will give them better protection. People who have something wrong with them understand that their immune system has failed them.

I'd make a terrible doctor. You see, if I had just diagnosed someone sitting in front of me as having a cancer I'd be saying, *'Right, before I send you off for surgery, radiotherapy or chemotherapy, let's sort out two things:*

Firstly, what might have caused your cancer – and so could still be there maintaining it. We'll then do our best to remove the threat.

Secondly, let's do everything in our power to re-boot your immune system so it is as strong as possible, before you have any debilitating orthodox therapies'.

While the full answer to this first question may be beyond the scope of this book, I hope that by now you feel that food, natural compounds and 'good diet' can correct causes like 'poor diet', some infections and even some toxins. And where it cannot correct, it could well hold the symptoms at bay.

Eat a spectrum of Rainbow Foods – and supplement

A summary:

1. **The liver** is the organ of detoxification in the body and in cancer patients it becomes toxic. To recap:

   - Fats and cholesterol 'clog it up' anyway.
   - There may be dead bacteria, microbes or even parasites.
   - The cholesterol can collect around dead cells and form gall-stones – there may be thousands of these particles, most

255

only the size of grains of sand. One US estimate was that 99.99 per cent of cancer patients had gallstones blocking the bile ducts so the liver could not excrete the toxins into the waste system properly.

- Then there is the lactic acid from cancer cells. Plus the drugs from steroids to chemotherapy that must be detoxified. And then there may be lots of dead cancer cells.

You need to strengthen your liver – milk thistle, magnesium will help
You need to clean it out – a detox of olive oil and Epsom Salts should do the trick.
And you need to dilate the bile ducts to enhance excretion of toxins – boldo tea, artichoke and dandelion will help. As will a series of coffee enemas.

2. **Exercise** improves the immune system. It moves the lymph to take toxins away from cells, it oxygenates the blood, and it increases levels of happy endorphins and Human Growth Hormone, both of which can reduce levels of 'bad hormones'. Research shows that half an hour every day is the level you need – if you can manage it. It does not have to be strenuous.

3. **Sunshine** can boost the immune system because it causes the production of vitamin D from cholesterol under your skin. Cancer cells have greater numbers of vitamin D receptor sites that normal cells – it kills them. And it boosts your whole immune system. If you cannot get 30 minutes in the sunshine everyday, take a supplement of 1000-2000 IU's of vitamin D3.

4. **Antioxidants**

    A) Research shows that vegetables and fruit provide more antioxidants from their natural compounds than are derived from synthetic vitamin supplements – providing you EAT WHOLE FOODS and that they are ORGANIC.

    Top natural food sources for the everyday antioxidants are:

Vitamin E: 2 tablespoons of sunflower seeds (11 mgs); 20 almonds (8 mgs); 1 tablespoon wheat germ (3mgs).

Vitamin C: 1 large red pepper (224 mgs); 100 gms raw broccoli (90 mgs) 150 gms papaya (90 mgs); 1 large orange (65 mgs).

Beta-carotene: 1 cup carrot juice (24 mgs); 1 medium sweet potato (10.0 mgs) 5 dried apricots (6.2 mgs); 1 cup cherries (6.2 mgs); half cup cooked spinach (5.7 mgs).

Zinc: 6 oysters (55 mgs), I medium steak (8 mgs); 4 tablespoons sunflower seeds (96mgs); serving of All Bran (4 mgs).

Selenium: 4 cracked Brazil nuts (150 mcgs); 4 slices of wholemeal bread (60 mcgs); 2 tablespoons sunflower seeds (15 mcgs); 1 free range egg (15 mcgs); 1 chicken breast (10 mcgs).

Lycopene: Tomatoes – 1 tin tomato soup (65 mgs); 5 tablespoons tomato paste (22 mgs).

B) The major problem with trying to 'Eat your vitamins and minerals' is that soil depletion has caused big losses. The US Government Senate has reviewed the matter three times and each time concluded that people should supplement. Especially with minerals. Vitamin E research with cancer uses levels of 200 mgs – from the above figures you will see that achieving these levels is almost impossible simply by eating. As always we only recommend taking natural compounds as supplements.

Supplements:

(i)   **Minerals:**

Zinc: 15 mgs per day

Selenium: 200 mcgs per day

(ii) **Vitamins:**

Vitamin E – Natural 8 forms, **Total Vitamin E** – 400 IU's per day

Vitamin B-12 and beta-carotene (plus many others) take **Chlorella** three times daily with meals

Coenzyme Q10: 30-50 mgs per day

C) **Eat RAINBOW FOODS:** The breakthrough in very recent times has been the discovery of natural compounds like **flavenoids and phenols** in plants, which are many, many times more powerful as antioxidants than 'bog standard' vitamin supplements. So 'Eat a Rainbow': A rainbow of colour and foods from red peppers, raspberries, pomegranates and cherries; to oranges, papaya and apricots; to yellow pinapples, grapefruit, ginger and nuts; to greens, onions, apples; to blues and red-purples like beetroot, plums, figs, aubergines. And, yes, there are some supplements you can add to this like:

Resveratrol: As directed on pack
Grape seed extract: As directed on pack
Curcumin (Turmeric): 2x 400 mgs per day
Take **bee propolis**, or eat Manuka Honey.

D) The next scientific breakthough has been the discovery of the importance of polysaccharides in boosting the levels of T-and B- lymphocytes, cytokines, interleukin and Natural Killer cells. Medicinal mushrooms (Shiitake, Reishi, cordyceps) have been used in the Far East in this way for years.

Top immune polysaccharide boosters are:

Aloe Vera: Sip a capful at night on retiring, and first thing in the morning

MGN-3 (Biobran): As directed on pack

D-Mannose: As directed on pack (also available in Ambrotose)

And the herbs:

Echinacea: Use tincture – depends on concentration – as directed

Cat's Claw: Use tincture – depends on concentration – as directed

Astragalus: Use tincture – depends on concentration – as directed

The last three we used with great effect after chemotherapy drugs had reduced my daughter's white cell count to low levels and the immune stimulating drugs were having no effect.

5. **Take a multi-strain Probiotic:** Beneficial Bacteria are the directors of the immune system. Over 1000 research studies and 80 clinical trials in the last 6 years have shown that they are essential ingredients for a strong immune system.

   Take:

   Neways Advanced Probiotic; Prebiota 7, and *L. Shirota* is only available in **Yakult.**

6. **Take notable others!**
   As we have covered before inflammation and possible microbial action cause your immune system to weaken. As insurance take:

   Fish Oils: As directed on pack

   Garlic supplement (if you can't eat 4 bulbs a day!): As directed on pack

7. **Eat potassium and magnesium-rich foods** – do not eat sugar or salt. Sugar weakens your immune system, smoothies are the worst! Salt causes your cells to become acid. Your cells and immune system work best when they are alkaline, and that means lots of potassium and magnesium-rich foods most of which are within our Rainbow Foods list: like lentils, pulses, jacket potato, nuts, whole grains and 'greens', bananas, whole brown rice, carrots, apples, pears, papaya and melon.

8. **Laugh** – laughter boosts the immune system and moves your

lymph. So see friends, watch old movies you like, old comedy shows, and go and see a show. Cut all the people and things out of your life that make you feel guilty, stressed or depressed. Let no-one put you down.

CHAPTER 26
FOOD FOR THOUGHT

Cooking tips

Although many books extol the benefits of raw food, others believe juicing helps to break up cellular structures and release minerals and enzymes. Some believe lightly cooking, even blanching, helps digestion and absorption. Too many cooks wash the vitamins away with the boiled water.

Roasting is the next best route providing that little, if any, fat is used, and items are slowly roasted with oven temperature below 120°C, especially for potatoes to avoid acrylamides. Please watch the fat content.

Wood or coal barbecues are poor ideas: Smoke and flames burn the meat and increase levels of highly carcinogenic nitrosamines. Use an electric grill, or 'fake' charcoal (but it's really gas) grill. Best to grill by wrapping the fish in foil before putting it on the barbecue.

Fried food is linked to higher rates of hormonally driven cancers in women, and men who eat fried food regularly have a three-fold increase in cancer. Who needs the fats and oils, the insulin and oestrogen surges and the dangerous free-radicals?

Microwaves polarise general opinion but not mine! In one study, Kirlian photography (which shows the energetic forces naturally occurring around a body or a plant) showed a strong field around broccoli both in its raw state and after steaming – but absolutely no energetic aura after just one second in a microwave. Every atom in every molecule in your food has electrons spinning in specific defined ways. In a microwave the atoms are energised to heat the food and it is absolutely impossible to expect all the electrons to be in the places they should have been when you turn off the microwave. You are eating irradiated, genetically modified food. William Kopp studies German and Russian papers on the subject and concluded that microwaved food is nutritionally deficient, and increases the number of

261

cancerous cells circulating in the bloodstream. Beware, some restaurant chains only serve microwaved foods. Many restaurants use microwaves to defrost food.

Stews are actually full of nourishment. They are slow-cooked and the temperature is lower than would allow nitrosamines or acrylamides to form. The problem is fat levels.

'Woked food' is a trendy European idea of how South East Asians cook. They only do it in cities – it is not how they eat in the villages. Keep the oil to a minimum. (In Asia water and oyster, or fish sauce are actually used, not oil.) Vegetables are served crisper and retain higher nourishment values.

Eating tips

- Eat 5-6 meals a day – not one or two big ones. 'Graze' don't stuff.
- Prepare some healthy snacks in the morning to eat during the day – sliced vegetable to dip in olive oil/balsamic dressing; or a bowl of sunflower, pumpkin, sesame and linseeds with a few chopped nuts.
- Eat some raw vegetables as a snack about 20 minutes before you eat your lunch or dinner. Your hormones will then tell you to feel less hungry when you come to the main meal and you absorb up to 40 per cent more vitamins and minerals by eating them this way.
- Don't drink water shortly before, during or after the meal – you don't need to. And it will dilute your digestive enzymes and reduce your nourishment.
- Eat slowly and think about the food – don't watch TV or read the paper – you will eat too fast.
- Food is for enjoyment – it is not fuel.
- If you ever say, 'I'm starving', you are ill. No one in their home in the Western world knows what 'starving' is.
- Chew well or the carbohydrates will not be digested – they need the ptyalin from your saliva glands. If you don't digest your carbohydrates properly you will not get full nourishment, and you will constipate.
- Only put food that is whole in your mouth. Your body deserves nothing less.

- Eat less than you need to fill you up. Your stomach will tighten after a couple of days and you will eat less.
- If you feel hungry, drink a glass of water. You will fill up.
- If you believe you may have yeasts, fruit should always be consumed first, at the start of the meal and on an empty stomach, if at all. Otherwise it can sit on top of a meal and ferment. People on anti-yeast diets need to avoid this complication as the fermentation aids the growth of yeasts. Very sweet fruits are also to be avoided in this scenario. For healthy people without a yeast problem fruits may be eaten at any time.
- Vegetables, pulses and oats, for example, contain soluble fibre. This is essential to the alimentary canal where it dissolves, transports and helps excrete toxins and excess hormones. Organic, whole, brown rice should be eaten regularly as it is particularly good at cleansing your system.
- Green tea (especially decaffeinated) is a strong antioxidant and helps to balance any acidity in the food you have eaten. Red wine has similar benefits. It's OK to drink a glass of red wine!
- Do not eat carbohydrate and protein at the same time. In the wild, our natural environment saw us find tubers and eat them, or gorge at a fruit tree, or capture an animal. We didn't take them all back to the cave and eat them on the same plate. Your digestive system is not designed for this total simultaneous consumption.

Let me explain: The carbohydrate and ptyalin mixture passes to the stomach where it needs an alkaline environment for maximum efficiency. Carbohydrate on its own clears the stomach in about one hour. Protein on the other hand passes to the stomach where it meets its digestive enzyme pepsin and this requires an acid environment. Protein on its own can be digested in about one and a half hours.

But mix the two and the stomach doesn't know whether to be alkaline or acid, with the result that the food is improperly digested and takes up to eight hours to pass through. This results in inefficiency throughout the intestinal system. It is also further hampered in the over 50s who anyway produce less acid.

It is particularly important to people over 50 that they avoid mixing protein and carbohydrate on the same fork! Levels of acid in the stomach can anyway decline by 30 per cent after 50 making digestion and absorption of key vitamins a problem.

Meal making tips

- Get planting – why not plant some fruit trees in a sunny area? Wisley Royal Gardens have fruit trees for all sizes of gardens.
- Grow some vegetables and fruits yourself. Runner beans, perpetual spinach, gooseberries, raspberries are all very easy.
- Have a little herb garden – you can even do this in pots on a patio or balcony.
- Sprout some seeds – buy Mung beans, or even broccoli seeds and put them in a covering of water on a little tray for three days in the window.
- Find a supplier of organic meat – chicken, game and so on.
- Eat more spices – flavor vegetables with turmeric, or saffron.
- Eat more salads – can you grow your own? Add olive oil or walnut oil – throw out the mayonnaise.
- Make your own breakfast muesli from whole grains, dried fruits, organic sunflower seeds, pumpkin seeds, crushed pecan nuts and a few psyllium seeds or linseeds.
- Find a supplier of organic fruit and vegetables.
- Make your own bread without refined wheat, sugar or salt.
- Buy a good juicer and make your own juices using nourishing vegetables and fruit like carrots, ginger, and apples.
- Buy a reverse osmosis water filter to provide water for cooking and washing utensils.
- Talk to the local restaurant and try to get the phone number of a supplier of glass bottled mineral water for drinking.
- Make your own nourishing soups.

CHAPTER 27

THE RAINBOW DIET:
EATING A SPECTRUM OF BENEFITS

The Ten Truths

From the outset I have told you ten truths about cancer:

1. Your cancer is as individual as you are – there are many causes.
2. It is not an item – it is a process.
3. It has many stages, many facets.
4. There will never be a magic bullet that can tackle all the causes and stages, simultaneously.
5. For thousands of years we have developed 'illnesses' throughout the day. Our inbuilt body systems are usually strong enough to correct and heal them.
6. This illness and healing struggle doesn't stop the moment a doctor tells you that you have cancer.
7. The factors that caused a cancer could still be maintaining it.
8. Also your defences are almost certainly weakened, and unable to cope.
9. The principles of prevention and correction are much the same – but the major difference is that there are less steps to tackle in prevention, more to tackle when correcting.
10. A multi-step development process demands a multi-step programme to tackle it.

The width of natural compounds

In my humble opinion, the only potential multi-stage protective and corrective programme involves a spectrum of natural compounds in food – unless someone in power somewhere is contemplating cancer patients taking 50 different drugs to combat 50 different possible causes and steps in the cancer process! Only food and natural compounds have the width to tackle all the steps necessary to both protect and correct. Only food and natural compounds have the spectrum of benefits capable of delivering. Only food and natural compounds have the ability to be used in combination and volume without side-effects or debilitating consequences. And finally many natural compounds seem to have a synergistic effect enhancing the effect of each other and often following different pathways to healing.

And before professors rush to put pen to paper in Medical Journals, or overweight nurses think to throw more books at us, please remember that many microbiologists and biochemists in universities and pharmaceutical companies at this very moment are actively working on natural compounds and trying to make synthetic versions they can patent and therefore profit from. I can list any number of natural compounds that are being concentrated and reformulated right now – from vitamin D to quercitin – how many do you want?

The pharmaceutical companies know that natural compounds are capable of repairing damaged DNA, reducing levels of bad oestrogen, preventing tumour formation and even killing cancer cells. They know they can help their drugs identify cancer cells, help the immune system identify cancer cells and even help reduce side effects.

So what's the big deal? Eminent professors will agree that a 'Good Diet' will prevent cancer. Why won't the same people own up to the fact that a spectrum of natural compounds that covers all the bases can be protective and corrective, if you can eat enough of them?

But what is enough? Already we have seen that just one glass of organic red wine a day has a significant effect, and half a cup of raspberries. Preventing, and correcting.

Let us change the paradigm. When research on natural compounds takes place it nearly always studies just one ingredient – at best a couple of vitamins. And that's why when studies on high doses of vitamin C in Arizona show that a number of cancer cells have their oxygen levels increased and it kills them, orthodox medical 'experts' rush to belittle the findings and the compounds by saying, '*It's not a cure for cancer*'.

No it isn't – but then nor is Herceptin, or Tamoxifen.

266

Let's get it clear for the final time – to effectively beat cancer – whether preventing or healing – you need width. You need a spectrum. You need a rainbow of natural compounds, to work together and cover all the bases. Vitamin C used as part of a much bigger package will do a job.

In my view natural compounds

- are easier to obtain,
- are much cheaper,
- have few or no side effects,
- have been through clinical trials for 200,000 years,
- have the necessary WIDTH to do the job.

A multi-step programme?

In Chapter 1 I told you that I would show you how a spectrum of natural compounds could tackle the various stages of cancer – protecting and correcting. Healing the daily illnesses. Let's see if I have done this.

* **Providing important factors to perfect DNA copying**

For example: Folic acid (Sources: leafy green vegetables, avocado, pulses, carrots, apricots) is able to help here.

For example: Anthocyanins protect the DNA and reduce copying errors (Sources: Purple colour foods like beetroot, blackcurrants, dark olives, elderberry, figs, deep red plums, red grapes, blueberries, blackberries, aubergine, red onion, red cabbage).

* **Providing important factors to correct DNA mis-copying**

For example: Genistein promotes levels of repair proteins in cells.

For example: Resveratrol repairs and boosts repair genes (red grapes, blackberries).

For example: I have told you how bee propolis protects healthy DNA whilst helping attack cancer cells.

* **Avoiding excesses of factors that increase free radicals**

For example: I have told you how smoking, trans fats,

saturated fats, acrylamides, microwave cooking and other poor diet factors can cause increases in free radicals.
For example: I have told you about calorie control. And the effect of sirtuins and resveratrol.

* **Providing more antioxidants to neutralise free radicals**

   For example: I have told you that OPC's (pine bark, grape seed) are 20-50 times stronger antioxidants. They are also found in apples, pears and cranberries. Lemongrass is another powerful antioxidant.
   For example: I have told you about many natural compound antioxidants from curcumin to betan glucan polysaccharides in medicinal mushrooms, and Biobran. And the concentrate of most – propolis.

* **Removing the toxic chemicals and heavy metals from your body and cells**

   For example: I have told you of the benefits of beneficial bacteria in conjunction with chlorella and lignans.
   For example: I have told you about selenium.
   For example: I have told you about indoles and dioxin elimination.

* **Boosting your immune system and helping it 'see' rogue cells**

   For example: I have told you how the herbs echinacea and cat's claw can boost your white cells and how astragalus can help in this and make rogue cells more available to the immune system.
   For example: I have told you of the benefits of supplementation with multi-strain probiotics. And the effects of spirulina and chlorella on your white cells.

* **Keeping your cells and immune system alkaline**

   For example: I have told you have eating potassium and magnesium rich foods (lentils, whole potato, broad beans, peas, whole grains, nuts, bananas) and avoiding sodium foods can achieve this.

* **Avoiding parasite and microbial infection**

  For example: I have told you the natural compounds that can kill most parasites (cloves, wormwood herb, fennel, garlic).

  For example: I have told you the natural compounds that can kill *Helicobacter pylori* like goldenseal herb, curcumin and olive oil.

  For example: I have told you what natural compounds kill yeasts (coconut, garlic, oregano) and given you a diet.

* **Minimising pathogens in the blood stream**

  For example: I have told you about several natural compounds like quercitin, which is an natural antibiotic (onions, apples, honey)

  For example: Ellagic acid is anti-bacterial and anti-viral (Sources: pomegranate, raspberries, walnuts)

  For example: Pau D'Arco is anti-viral, anti-bacterial, anti-fungal.

* **Reducing inflammation – a precursor of many cancers**

  For example: I have told you how the COX-2 enzyme can be turned off by fish oils, aspirin, aloe vera, ginger and phenols, for example in olive oil and green tea

  For example: I have told you about the many active ingredients in bee propolis

* **Preventing a blood supply to the developing tumour**

  For example: I have told you the benefits of sulphur compounds like sulphoraphanes and garlic; and also about isoflavones.

* **Lowering aggressive oestradiol levels**

  For example: I have told you about indoles (Sources: Greens, cabbage, broccoli).

  For example: I have told you about melatonin and asphalia.

  For example: I have told you about phytoestrogens and genistein (Sources: red clover and pulses).

* **Keeping blood and cellular oxygen levels up**

For example: I have told you the benefits of regular daily exercise, supported by vitamin C and especially foods that contain glutathione (Sources: most fruits and vegetables especially green ones).

* **Strengthening your liver, and therefore your immune system**

For example: I have told about the benefits of a liver flush using Epsom Salts and olive oil.

For example: I have told you the benefits of magnesium, soya lecithin, and of coffee enemas and of the herbs boldo and dandelion in the elimination of toxins.

* **Increasing your pancreatic enzyme production**

For example: I have told you about chromium picolinate and about a low glycaemic/whole food diet.

* **Killing cancer cells**

For example: I have told you about nitrilosides (Sources: bitter natural foods like quince, almonds, macadamia nuts, gooseberries, papaya, bamboo shoots, yams and sprouting seeds).

For example: I have told you about research on chapperal; on capsaicin (Source: chilli peppers) and on sulphoraphanes (Source: sprouting seeds)

For example: I have told you about quercitin and its ability to heat up cancer cells and kill them.

* **Increases survival rates**

For example: I have told you about the big research studies – the China Study and Su.Vi Max studies on antioxidants vitamin E, C, beta carotene and zinc and selenium and how they reduce mortality from cancer.

In fact I've told you about much more than this – about the wonderful width of benefits that natural compounds have – but do not forget the great reduction fertilisers, pesticides and herbicides have on their levels.

A fundamental truth

We've seen that the diet therapies of Gonzalez, Pfeifer and Gerson are quite rigorous and disciplined. They cover all the bases. John Boik did exactly that too – perfect if you want that sort of detail.

But the rest of us are just ordinary folk trying in our own ways to get a little discipline into our diets, and give ourselves the very best odds of beating a cancer. And I believe the answer is exactly the same as these professionals employ – and that is width. A discipline that is simple to use, and goes right across the many stages of cancer.

And for this reason I am far more in favour of the French Diet with hints of the Macrobiotic discipline than the Vegetarian, South East Asian, or whatever. For me the French Diet, and particularly the Mediterranean Diet, has a corrective enormity. It also acknowledges a fundamental truth that comes out of the studies on these natural compounds. And that is that there are foods around us, in our local environments, that we have eaten fresh and in season for thousands of years, **and they work with our bodies to protect and correct us all day long.** They heal our illnesses.

In a normal week we no longer consume:

* Radishes, red peppers and raspberries.
* Turmeric, oranges and honey.
* Onions, fresh nuts, ginger and limes.
* Spinach, broccoli, watercress, Brussel sprouts and quince.
* Oily fish, clean water.
* Beetroot, cherries, pomegranate.
* Blackberries, seeds and figs.
* Herbs like oregano, marjoram, sage and thyme.

And this is why I find the Government's standard of *'Eat 5 portions of fruit and vegetables a day'*, completely meaningless. Most people think that means you can have chips three times and tomato sauce on your pizza.

The issue is width – the solution is a spectrum – and the delivery is The Rainbow Diet.

271

CHAPTER 28
THE RAINBOW DIET:
THE SHOPPING TROLLEY

Some core 'rules'

First read out loud:

1. I will try to avoid salt and sugar, and processed and packaged foods.
2. I will try to avoid dairy.
3. I will try to avoid fizzy soft drinks, fruit juices and smoothies, sweeteners and refined products.
4. I will only put whole foods in my mouth.
5. I will supplement – but I will only use natural supplements.
6. I will grow more of my own foods.
7. I will eat more fresh foods; living foods – especially those that are locally grown and in season.
8. I will try to find a supplier I can trust to supply organic food.
9. I will only drink clean water.
10. I will fill my kitchen and my plate each week with the colours of the Rainbow.

Be inspired. There is so much to choose from and to enjoy.

Eat a Rainbow

No longer will you struggle to eat 5 portions of fruit and vegetables a day. Instead you are going to have two large flat plates or bowls sitting in your kitchen – one of vegetables and the other of fruit. And each is going to have a rainbow of wonderful colours in them.

Reds for ellagic acid, resveratrol and lycopene, deep purples for anthocyanins, orange for carotenoids, yellow for honey and propolis, blues for pterostilbene, greens for polyphenols, indoles, and vitamin K, apples and onions for quercitin, herbs for their cancer killing powers and more. All washed down by a glass of red wine or a cup of green tea.

Research from Ohio State University has shown that these positive natural compounds have more effect, the more you eat. And research from Illinois University has shown that these natural compounds frequently affect different anti-cancer enzyme pathways. Eat lots of different colours and lots of each colour. And take a daily dose of sunshine (30 minutes should be enough) and drink clean water.

The shopping trolley

The best way to plan your healthy diet is to prevent yourself being weak-willed. Pre-plan and only bring healthy foods into your home. *"It is not the mountains we conquer, but ourselves"*, according to Sir Edmund Hillary. Sometimes we just need a little help towards that self-discipline.

Now I realise not all of these products are from the UK and locally grown but I wanted you to see a real width of possible products so you could choose for yourself. Here is a look at what your shopping trolley can contain:

RED:

Red peppers, tomatoes, tomato puree, pomegranates, raspberries, strawberries, red currants, cranberries, radish, red grapes, chilli peppers, watermelon.

ORANGE:

Oranges, apricots, peaches, turmeric, carrots, mangoes, papaya, yams, bananas, satsumas, clementines.

YELLOW:

Garlic, ginger, oats, onions, saffron, yellow peppers, fresh sweetcorn, squash, bamboo shoots, lemons, limes, melon, pineapple, nectarines, grapefruit, honey. Nuts – fresh Brazil, pecan, macadamia, walnuts, cashews.

GREEN:

Watercress, spinach, broccoli, greens, cabbage, kale, Brussel sprouts, chard, courgettes, avocados, green tea, fennel, green beans, runner beans, cauliflower, celery, apples, pears, asparagus tips, chives, spring onions, cucumber, lettuce, endive, leeks, green peppers, broad beans, peas, sprouting seeds, alfalfa, plums, green grapes, kiwi fruit.

PURPLE:

Aubergines, red plums, figs, beetroot, blackberries, blueberries, blackcurrants, lentils, red kidney beans, wild and brown rice, Japanese mushroom, pumpkin seeds, cherries, dates.

WHITE/BROWN:

Oats, barley, buckwheat, millet, rye, clean water, potatoes, onions, parsnips, turnips, garlic, whole grain pasta, sunflower seeds, sesame seeds, psyllium seeds, lychees, swede, butter beans, chick peas, hummus, coconut milk, deep-sea caught fish, oysters, rice milk, soya milk, goat's milk, eggs, wheatgerm*.

HERBS and SPICES: Mint, sorrel, sage, thyme, coriander, nutmeg, cinnamon, lemon grass, saffron.

OILS: Extra virgin olive oil, walnut oil.

OTHER: Dried fruits, Quorn, red wine (Cabernet Sauvignon is best – especially organic), apricot kernels, eat the grape seeds.

REGULAR SUPPLEMENTS

Prebiota 7; Neway's Advanced Probiotic
Chlorella (better than spirulina or wheatgrass)
Fish oils
Total (all 8 forms) vitamin E
Coenzyme Q10
Selenium
Zinc
Aloe vera
Resveratrol
Grape seed extract

Vitamin D3
Turmeric/curcumin
Quality mineral supplement
Occasional herbs – like astragalus, echinacea, cat's claw

(*You may prefer to avoid wheat)

CHAPTER 29

THE RAINBOW DIET:
THE PROGRAMME

The Programme

The aim is to keep it simple.

The target is 100 points per day (especially for those with cancer). Eat what you want but beat the target, everyday. Have fun.

Daily Starting Score

This is your start point each day. You can get a head start if you watch out for the following:

1) If you do 30 minutes 'exercise' every day
   award yourself: + 15 points
2) If you filter your tap water with a reverse
   osmosis filter, and drink glass bottled water: + 15 points
3) If you sleep in a completely darkened room: + 5 points
4) If you are correct weight for your height: + 5 points
5) If you are 4kgs overweight: – 3 points
6) If you are 10kgs overweight: – 20 points
7) If you smoke at all: – 20 points
8) If you take a daily Probiotic multi-strain
   supplement: + 5 points
9) If the majority of your food is organic: + 10 points
10) If you have 30 minutes of sunshine – or
   supplement with vitamin D3 (1000 IU's): + 5 points

Points for foods

All points have been assigned on a balance basis. For example, baked beans have the benefits of tomato (puree) and pulses, but the negatives of lots of sugar and salt and being canned.

Whole grain pasta is beneficial and achieves a positive score. Normal pasta is worthless.

Fresh is best

Give yourself 3 points extra if you eat something organic, although strictly speaking, everything you eat should be organic.

This is meant to be a fun programme, so we have not assigned detailed weights or volumes.

The principle is that you can have your piece of lamb, if you really enjoy it, but put a tomato stuffed with garlic and parsley with it; perhaps some unrefined wild rice and lentils. This is how you pick up points and how you add in protective agents and eat to beat cancer.

It's not an ingredient but the totality of the meal that matters.

10 Points (1 serving e.g. large serving spoon)

FRESH, LOCALLY GROWN VEGETABLES AND FRUIT (LOW GI)

Alfalfa and sprouting seeds	Leeks
Apples	Lettuce (various)
Apricots	Olives
Asparagus tips	Onions
Berries	Parsnips
Beetroot	Peaches
Cabbage	Pears
Cauliflower	Pomegranates
Celery	Raspberries
Chard	Radishes
Cherries	Redcurrants
Chives	Spring onions
Cucumber	Sorrel
Endive	Spinach
Garlic (1 clove raw)	Squash
Ginger	Swede
Green beans	Tomatoes
Kale	Turnip
Kelp	Watercress

10 Points (continued)

FRESH NUTS
e.g. Almonds
  Brazils
  Cashews
  Pecans
  Macadamia nuts
  Walnuts

PULSES
e.g. Broad beans
  Butter beans
  Chickpeas
  Kidney beans
  Lentils
  Peas

SEEDS
Pumpkin
Sesame
Sunflower
(N.B. Alcohol outside meal score -5)

DRINKS
1–2 glasses red wine
especially Cabernet
Sauvignon with meal

OILS
Flaxseed oil
Linseed oil (linseeds)

FLESH
Deep-sea caught oily fish

CARBOHYDRATE AND GRAINS
Fresh boiled potato
Brown unrefined rice, wild rice
Oats, millet, barley, buckwheat
Unrefined grains

OTHER
Home-made muesli
Home-pressed fruit juices

5 Points

IMPORTED FRUITS AND VEGETABLES AND DRIED FRUITS
e.g. Avocados
  Bamboo shoots
  Bananas
  Cranberries
  Currants and raisins
  Dates
  Dried fruits
  Figs
  Grapes
  Spicy chillies

5 Points cont'd

Lemons
Lychees
Mangoes
Melon
Papaya
Peppers
Satsumas
Yams

OTHERS

Aloe vera
Eggs – poached, boiled (free range and organic)
Garlic (cooked)

HERBS

Basil, fennel, coriander
Home-made bread (no salt, sugar – add seeds)
Honey
Hummus
Japanese mushrooms – e.g. Reishi, Maiitake, Cordyceps
Psyllium seeds
Spices – turmeric, chilli, cinnamon, nutmeg, saffron
Supermarket high grade muesli, or non-baked cereals

FLESH

Locally caught oily fish

2 Points

OTHER

Baked potato
Canned fish
Canned fruit
Coconut milk
Green tea – 1 cup
Natural oat bran
Organic lean chicken, turkey, game (max 1 serving per day. Any further serving – 5 points.)

2 Points cont'd

Potatoes (fresh) or mashed (no milk)
Quorn Soups (chilled)
Soya and soy milk
Spices – chilli, cinnamon and nutmeg Sweetcorn Tomato puree
(not ketchup)

OTHER FRUITS
1 orange (max. per day)

0 Points

Bagels
Baked beans
Herb teas
Jams
Marmalade
Muesli bars, cereal bars
Organic bread
Organic meat, poultry, game
Processed fruit juices
Shoyu and tamari soy sauce
Smoked fish
Soups

0 Points cont'd

Stir-frying
Sunflower, safflower oils
Tomato ketchup
White wine
Wholemeal bread

–5 Points

Alcopops
Any processed food, ready meals (e.g. instant noodles, packaged
soups), frozen meals
Beer, spirits, liqueurs
Biscuits
Bread, waffles – white or malted
Cakes

−5 Points cont'd

Chips
Chocolate snack products
Coffee
Crispbreads
Crisps, peanuts (salted)
Fizzy soft drinks
Mayonnaise
Pasta
Pizza
Processed breakfast cereals
Refined wheat, grains, sugar, rice
Rice cakes
Salt
Smoked meats
Sweeteners
Tea

−10 Points

Any dairy/milk product/yoghurts
Bacon, pepperoni, frankfurters, sausages, dried meats, pâté, rilletes
Barbecued food
Fast food (e.g. burgers, chicken portions, chips)
Fried foods
Hydrogenated vegetable oils
Margarines
Microwaved food
Pickled foods
Chinese foods

CHAPTER 30
THE RAINBOW DIET: A POSTSCRIPT

'Food colours could hold the key to new cancer drugs'

Thus ran the heading in a UK Newspaper recently. Let me quote you Dr Monica Giusti, from Ohio State University in Columbus. 'All fruits and vegetables that are rich in anthocyanins have compounds that can slow down the growth of cancer cells'. She went on to suggest that synthetic food dyes should be replaced by the use of anthocyanin-based pigments instead. What a good idea.

In a number of research studies at Ohio, experiments using a variety of foods have shown that cancer cell growth could be 'significantly' reduced and foods with the highest levels of active ingredients were most effective – what a surprise!

Scientists are now investigating concentrating the chemicals to provide a 'new generation of drugs'.

A search of the research shows that this is already happening with:

Anthocyanins – where companies are looking at their use in killing cancer cells.

Indoles – where Companies want to reduce levels of aggressive oestrogen, block receptor sites on cells and neutralise by-products of oestrogen.

Polyphenols – where companies are looking at how they can repair DNA; and how they can kill rogue cells.

Polysaccharides – where companies are looking at how they can improve communications between cells, especially enhancing the immune system to recognise and attack cancer cells.

Astragalus – where companies are looking at how it can expose cancer cells to be recognised by the immune system.

Feverfew and some 18 other herbs – where companies are

looking to isolate the active ingredient and concentrate it to kill cancer cells.

Vitamin D – has now been concentrated and is in stage III of Clinical Trials, showing huge potential

Wormwood and Pau D'Arco – both being studied for their active anti-viral ingredients.

Capsaicin – being studied for its ability to kill cancer cells directly.

Resveratrol – being studied for its ability to replicate calorie restriction benefits in the body, repair DNA and treat Alzheimer's to brain tumours.

And probably a hundred more.

While the Pharmaceutical Companies are concentrating these natural compounds you can be eating the benefits, today. And anyway, if they are herbs, concentrates already exist – they are called tinctures.

The truth is that the Pharmaceutical Companies, through their actions are clearly endorsing the benefits of these natural compounds – they deliver.

Why wait for the synthetic versions? You can start eating the powerful, organic natural versions of these compounds today. And the more you eat the greater the effect.

'Eating different natural compounds multiplies the effect'

The University of Illinois has been studying lycopene (from tomatoes) and indole-3-carbinol (from broccoli). Each is known to have a positive benefit with prostate cancer. John Erdman, Professor of Food Science says that they are quite different substances and don't have to be eaten together to have an effect. But when combined, there effect seems to multiply up. They work on completely different anti-cancer pathways, but eating both in the same meal seems to have a much greater effect.

Better than drugs – is another myth going to bite the dust?

In the same studies, Erdman concluded that the combined effect of broccoli and tomatoes had better results than the oestrogen inhibitor Finasteride.

But then indole-3-carbinol is producing better results than Tamoxifen, Pterostilbene produced better results than cipofibrate, ellagic acid was better than HPV preventing drugs, and the herb Feverfew produced better results than the leukaemia drug cytarabine. I could list many more. All this, when we are repeatedly told that drugs need to be formulated to concentrate the active ingredient and give it more power – I believe the answer to this is another natural compound, rhubarb!

Interestingly, Christie Manchester has a novel way of treating infections of the mouth and throat after chemo and radiotherapy. No more are they thinking of providing drugs. Instead they are turning to the natural anti-bacterial powers of Manuka honey.

Eat a rainbow

So what are you waiting for? Go on, 'Eat a Rainbow' – take some sunshine into your life, add some quality supplements from the list, drink clean water, look for organic fruits and vegetables from a good local supplier – and even grow a few yourself. Now, enjoy a long life of protection.

I am absolutely convinced from everything I have read in the last 6 years and in preparing this book that natural compounds are an essential part of any prevention or treatment programme and offer everybody a real opportunity to correct and heal.

Liver Cleanse / Gallstone Flush

Ingredients:

½ cup extra virgin olive oil
1 very big grapefruit (providing ¾ cup of juice)
4 tablespoons of Epsom Salts
3 cups of water
Ornithine tablets.

Preparation:

Set aside 3 days.

Day 1:

Eat a no-fat breakfast and lunch.
Eat and drink nothing after 2.00 pm.
Mix the Epsom Salts in the water (easier if water is warm), then cool.

6.00 pm	Drink a quarter of this liquid.
8.00 pm	Drink a further quarter of the liquid
10.00 pm	Mix the olive oil and pulp-free grapefruit juice and shake vigorously.
	Drink the liquid through a straw before 10.15 pm.
	Take four Ornithine tablets to help you sleep.
	Retire immediately and massage your stomach.
	Focus your mind on your liver and imagine the toxins leaving it, along with the stones.
	Sleep.

Day 2:

Upon waking and not before 7.00 am take the third quarter of the Epsom salts mix. Two hours later take the last quarter.

Expect diarrhoea for two days; don't eat before lunch time on day two and keep food to salads and fruit, plus baked potatoes for days two and three.

You may need to repeat this treatment after a few weeks. 2000–3000 small stones may be passed.

Please note – This recipe is derived from William Kelley's cancer treatment. It has thousands of testimonials, none report pain, only success; but nobody at **icon** has any first hand experience of it. And although a number of our readers have now tried the 'treatment' and been happy with the results, we are merely **told** it works!

FOR ALL THE INFORMATION

REGARDING CONTACT DETAILS

AND NATURAL SUPPLEMENTS IN

THIS BOOK, PLEASE RING

CANCERactive

ON 0203 186 1006

OR EMAIL

chris@canceractive.com

To order more copies of this book

Tel: 44(0)203 186 1006
Email: enquiries@canceractive.com

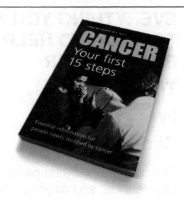

Our aim is to help people increase their personal odds of beating cancer by providing information – ALL the information – on complementary and alternative therapies not merely orthodox ones, so that people can make more informed choices.

We have a unique 2,000 page web site covering everything you need to know to help you beat cancer

We provide a unique quarterly magazine **icon** (Integrated Cancer and Oncology News) free to 370 UK cancer centres.

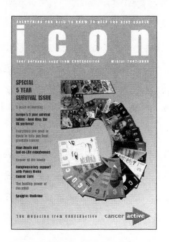

For more details contact us by email enquiries@canceractive.com; or by telephone 0203 186 1006.

CANCERactive
Intelligent Information. Independent Voice.